Professor Jennie Brand-Miller is Professor of Human Nutrition in the Human Nutrition Unit, School of Molecular and Microbial Biosciences at the University of Sydney, and President of the Nutrition Society of Australia. She has taught postgraduate students of nutrition and dietetics at the University of Sydney for over 25 years and currently leads a team of 12 research scientists. Professor Brand-Miller was recently awarded a Clunies Ross National Science and Technology Medal for her work in championing a new approach to nutrition and the management of blood glucose.

Kaye Foster-Powell is an accredited practising dietitian with extensive experience in diabetes management. A graduate of the University of Sydney (B.Sc., Master of Nutrition & Dietetics) she has conducted research into the glycaemic index of foods and its practical applications over the last 15 years. Currently she is the senior dietitian with Sydney West Diabetes Service and provides consultancy on all aspects of the glycaemic index.

Other books in the Low GI series

The Low GI Diet

The Low GI Diet Cookbook

Low GI Life Plan

The Low GI Guide to the Metabolic Syndrome and Your Heart

The Low GI Guide to Managing PCOS

Low GI Eating Made Easy

The New Glucose Revolution

The New Glucose Revolution & Children with Type 1 Diabetes

The New Glucose Revolution & Heavy Children

The New Glucose Revolution & Losing Weight

The New Glucose Revolution & Sports Nutrition

The New Glucose Revolution for People with Diabetes

The Low Gi

Shopper's Guide
to Gi Values

The glycaemic index
solution for optimum health

Dr Jennie Brand-Miller
the authority on low GI eating
and Kaye Foster-Powell

HODDER
MOBIUS

A huge thank you to Fiona Atkinson and other members of the
GI testing team (Anna, Marian, Kailyn).

Contents

Understanding the GI 1

   The GI explained 5

   Making the change to a low GI Diet 8

   Seven top tips for eating the healthy
low GI way 10

   Your daily food choices 11

   What to keep in your pantry 20

   What to keep in your refrigerator 23

   What to keep in your freezer 25

   How we calculate the GI 26

   Let's talk glycaemic load (GL) 28

   Look for the GI on the foods you buy 31

A to Z GI Values 33

Low to High GI Values 81

Understanding
the GI

If you want to change to a low GI diet or increase the amount of low GI food you are already eating, where do you start? Look no further than the *Shopper's Guide to GI Values*. Many foods today that have been tested by accredited laboratories display the authentic GI symbol. That part is easy. But what about other foods? With hundreds of foods—from breads and breakfast bars to fruit juice, fruit and vegetables—listed alphabetically, plus by category, this book will save you time in the supermarket by directing you to the best low GI foods available.

And you don't have to worry about giving up some of your favourite snacks or meals. Simply by swapping from one brand or type of food to another, you can improve the overall GI of your diet. This is where the tables in this book will become an essential part of your food shopping forever.

But first, what are the benefits of a low GI diet? There's no doubt that knowing the GI values of foods is your key to the enormous health benefits of *The New Glucose Revolution*.

Whether you are overweight, have diabetes, hypertension, elevated blood fats, heart disease or Syndrome X (the metabolic syndrome), you will benefit from eating a low GI diet. Or, if you want to do what you can to prevent these problems, you need to know about the glycaemic index of foods. You may consider you already eat a high-quality diet, but being aware of the GI values of foods is essential if you are interested in maintaining optimum health.

With that in mind, we've put together this handy guide full of GI values to help you put those low GI smart carb food choices into your shopping trolley and onto your plate. By doing so you'll satisfy your hunger, increase your energy levels and eliminate your desire to eat more than you should.

How to use the tables:
- if you want the actual GI value and glycaemic load (GL) of a food, turn to page 33 for a comprehensive A–Z listing of individual foods. We have cross-referenced this listing so you can check by brand name, food type or food category.
- if you want to know whether a food is high, medium or low GI, start on page 81 for our at-a-glance Low GI, Medium GI and High GI listings.

You can use the different listings to:
- find the GI of your favourite foods
- compare foods within a category (two types of bread, for example)
- improve your diet by finding a low GI substitute for high GI foods
- put together a low GI meal
- shop for low GI foods

If you can't find the GI value for a food you regularly eat, please write to the manufacturer and encourage them to have the food tested by an accredited laboratory such as Sydney University's Glycemic Index Research Service (SUGiRS). In the meantime, choose a similar food from the tables as a substitute.

The GI values in this book are correct at the time of publication. However, the formulation of commercial foods can change and the GI may change, too. You can rely on foods showing the GI symbol. Although some manufacturers include the GI value of their product on the label, you would need to know that the testing was carried out independently by an accredited laboratory, as represented by the authentic GI symbol (see page 31.)

The GI explained

Our research on the GI began more than 20 years ago—at about the time when health authorities around the world began to stress the importance of high-carbohydrate diets. Until then dietary fat had grabbed all the public and scientific attention, but low fat diets are by their very nature *automatically* high in carbohydrate. The rapidly rising numbers of people with obesity at this time led nutrition scientists to start asking questions— could carbohydrates be implicated in the development of obesity; are all carbohydrates the same; are all starches good for health and all sugars bad? To investigate, they began to study the effects of carbohydrates on blood glucose levels. They wanted to know which carbo- hydrate foods were associated with the least fluctuation in blood glucose levels and the best for overall health, including reduced risk of diabetes and heart disease.

Understanding the GI of foods helps you choose the right amount of carbohydrate and the right sort of carbohydrate for your long-term health and wellbeing.

The GI is a physiologically based measure of the effect carbohydrates have on blood glucose levels. It provides an easy and effective way to eat a healthy diet and at the same time control fluctuations in blood glucose.

- Carbohydrates that break down rapidly during digestion, releasing glucose quickly into the blood stream, have a high GI.

- Carbohydrates that break down slowly, releasing glucose into the blood stream gradually, have a low GI. We call these smart carbs.

> The rate of carbohydrate digestion has important implications for everybody. For most people, foods with a low GI have advantages over those with a high GI. They can:
> - improve blood glucose control
> - increase satiety as they are more filling and satisfying and reduce appetite
> - facilitate weight loss
> - improve blood fat profiles
> - reduce risks of developing diabetes, heart disease and certain types of cancer

A low GI diet has been scientifically proven to help people:
- with type 1 diabetes
- with type 2 diabetes
- with gestational diabetes (diabetes during pregnancy)
- who are overweight
- who have a normal weight but excess abdominal fat
- whose blood glucose levels are higher than desirable
- who have been told they have pre-diabetes, 'impaired glucose tolerance', or a 'touch of diabetes'
- with high levels of triglycerides and low levels of HDL-cholesterol ('good' cholesterol)

- with Syndrome X (the insulin resistance or metabolic syndrome)
- who suffer from polycystic ovarian syndrome (PCOS)
- who suffer from fatty liver disease (NAFLD or NASH)

If you would like to know more about the beneficial effects eating low GI foods can have on the above conditions, please refer to our other books in *The Low GI* series, a full list of which is shown at the beginning of this book.

Making the change to a low GI diet

Three things to remember:

1. The GI relates only to carbohydrate-rich foods

There are three main nutrients in food—protein, carbo-hydrate and fat. Meat, chicken, eggs and fish are high in protein; bread, rice, pasta and cereals are high in carbohydrate; and butter, margarine and oils are high in fat. We can only measure the GI of foods that contain carbohydrate.

2. The GI is not intended to be used in isolation

The GI value of a food alone does not make it good or bad for us. It is important to consider the overall nutritional value of a food, including the saturated fat, salt and fibre content—in addition to its GI value—when choosing foods for a balanced diet.

3. There is no need to eat only low GI foods

While most of us will benefit from eating low GI foods at each meal, this doesn't mean consuming these foods to the exclusion of all other carb foods. When we eat a combination of low and high GI carb foods, like baked beans on toast, fruit and sandwiches, lentils with rice, potatoes and corn, the final GI value of the meal is intermediate.

To get started, you need to:

EAT a lot more fruit and vegetables, pulses and wholegrain products such as barley and traditional oats.

PAY ATTENTION to breads and breakfast cereals—these foods contribute most to the glycaemic load of a typical British diet.

MINIMISE refined flour products and starches such as crumpets, crackers, biscuits, rolls and pastries, irrespective of their fat and sugar content.

AVOID high GI snacks such as pretzels, corn chips, rice cakes and crackers.

Seven top tips for eating the healthy low GI way

1. **Eat seven or more servings of fruit and vegetables every day (two fruit and five vegetables):** being high in fibre, and therefore filling, and low in fat (apart from olives and avocado, which contain 'good' fats), fruit and vegetables play a central role in low GI eating.

2. **Eat low GI breads and cereals:** the type of breads and cereals you eat affects the GI of your diet the most.

3. **Eat more pulses, including soyabeans, chickpeas and lentils**—nature's lowest GI foods.

4. **Eat nuts in small amounts regularly:** although nuts are high in fat (averaging around 50 per cent), it is largely unsaturated fat, so they make a healthy substitute for snacks such as biscuits, cakes, pastries, crisps and chocolate.

5. **Eat more fish and seafood.**

6. **Eat lean red meats, poultry and eggs:** these protein foods do not have a GI because they are not sources of carbohydrate. Red meat, however, is the best source of iron you can get.

7. **Eat low fat dairy foods:** milk, cheese, ice-cream, yoghurt, buttermilk and custard are the richest sources of calcium in our diet.

Your daily food choices

Three key habits to ensure a low GI diet

1. If you eat breakfast cereal, check out the GI of your favourite brand—you might get quite a surprise. Most of the popular big-name cereals have high GI values in the 70s and above.

2. Choose low GI bread. Steer clear of sweet biscuits, cakes, scones, doughnuts and bread rolls made from refined flour (except sourdough) as much as you can.

3. Eat fruit for at least one of your daily snacks and have a semi-skimmed milk drink or low fat yoghurt for another.

To help you achieve your *minimum* requirements for energy, protein, vitamins and minerals we have created two special GI food pyramids—one for Moderate Carb Eaters and one for Big Carb Eaters.

The recommended servings of each food group are shown with each pyramid. If you are a big bread and cereal eater, the GI pyramid for Big Carb Eaters will suit you best.

Either way, the serving information on pages 16–17 applies to both pyramids.

Healthy low GI diet tips
- Focus on what you eat, rather than what not to eat.
- Eat at least one low GI food at each meal.
- Reduce your intake of fat, especially saturated.
- Eat regularly; don't skip meals.

The GI Pyramid for Moderate Carb Eaters

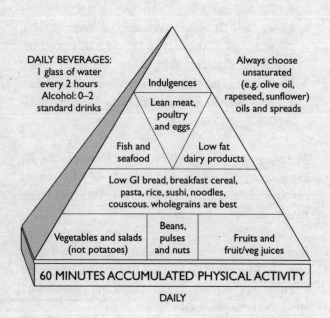

DAILY BEVERAGES:
I glass of water
every 2 hours
Alcohol: 0–2
standard drinks

Always choose
unsaturated
(e.g. olive oil,
rapeseed, sunflower)
oils and spreads

Indulgences

Lean meat,
poultry
and eggs

Fish and
seafood

Low fat
dairy products

Low GI bread, breakfast cereal,
pasta, rice, sushi, noodles,
couscous. wholegrains are best

Vegetables and salads
(not potatoes)

Beans,
pulses
and nuts

Fruits and
fruit/veg juices

60 MINUTES ACCUMULATED PHYSICAL ACTIVITY

DAILY

Daily food choices for Moderate Carb Eaters:

Indulgences: 1–2 servings

Fish and seafood/lean meat, poultry and eggs: 5–7 servings

Low fat dairy products: 2 servings

Bread, breakfast cereals, rice, pasta, noodles, grains: 4 servings

Vegetables and salads: 5 or more servings

Pulses: 1–2 servings

Fruit and juices: 1–3 servings

Nuts and oils: 2–4 servings

> The serving guidelines shown above are for the
> lowest recommended level of carbohydrate intake
> (40–45% of energy from carbohydrate) for a
> 1400–1900 calorie (6000–8000 kJ) diet. For the
> lower calorie intake, choose the smaller number of
> servings.

The GI Pyramid for Big Carb Eaters

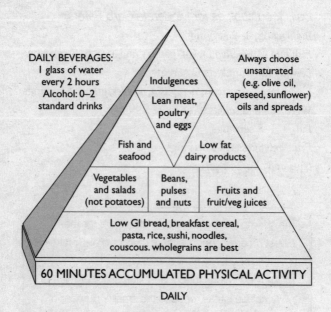

DAILY BEVERAGES:
I glass of water
every 2 hours
Alcohol: 0–2
standard drinks

Always choose
unsaturated
(e.g. olive oil,
rapeseed, sunflower)
oils and spreads

Indulgences

Lean meat,
poultry
and eggs

Fish and
seafood

Low fat
dairy products

Vegetables
and salads
(not potatoes)

Beans,
pulses
and nuts

Fruits and
fruit/veg juices

Low GI bread, breakfast cereal,
pasta, rice, sushi, noodles,
couscous. wholegrains are best

60 MINUTES ACCUMULATED PHYSICAL ACTIVITY

DAILY

Daily food choices for Big Carb Eaters:

Indulgences: 1–2 servings

Fish and seafood/lean meat, poultry and eggs: 3–5 servings

Low fat dairy products: 2 servings

Bread, breakfast cereals, rice, pasta, noodles, grains: 6–8
   servings

Vegetables and salads: 5 or more servings

Pulses: 1–2 servings

Fruit and juices: 3 servings

Nuts and oils: 2–3 servings

> The serving guidelines shown above are for an
> average carbohydrate intake (50–55% of energy
> from carbohydrate) for a 1400–1900 calorie (6000–
> 8000 kJ) diet. For the lower calorie intake, choose
> the smaller number of servings.

What's a serving?

Whether you eat carbs in moderate or large amounts, the portion sizes stay the same.

Indulgences

2 tablespoons (40 g) cream, sour cream

25 g chocolate

1 small slice (40 g) cake

1 small packet (30 g) crisps

2 standard alcoholic drinks* (1 standard drink is 100 ml wine, 30 ml spirits, 285 ml beer)

* National guidelines recommend an average daily limit of one standard alcoholic drink for women and two for men.

Fish, seafood, lean meats, poultry, eggs & alternatives

50 g (raw weight) boneless meat, fish or chicken

50 g canned fish

2 eggs

40 g reduced fat cheese or 30 g full fat cheese

100 g tofu

Pulses

½ cup cooked lentils, chickpeas, beans

Low fat dairy or alternative

1 cup (250 ml) milk or soya milk

200 g yoghurt

Nuts & oils
2 teaspoons olive or rapeseed oil
1 tablespoon oil-based vinaigrette
15 g nuts
40 g avocado

Breads, cereals, rice, pasta, noodles, grains
1 slice bread
½ cup cooked rice, pasta or noodles
½ cup (30 g) cereal

Fruit & juices
1 medium piece of fruit
1 cup small fruit pieces
½ cup (125 ml) juice

Vegetables
½ cup cooked vegetables
1 cup raw or salad vegetables

Making sense of food labelling

There's lots of information on food labels these days, but unfortunately, very few people know how to interpret it correctly. Often the claims on the front of the packet don't mean quite what you think. Here are some prime examples:

Cholesterol free—Take care, the food may still be high in fat.

Fat reduced—But is it low fat? Compare fat per 100 g between products.

No added sugar—Do you realise it could still raise your blood glucose?

Lite—Light in what? It could mean simply light in colour.

To get the hard facts on the nutritional value of a food, look at the Nutrition Information table. Here you'll find the details regarding the fat, calorie, carbohydrate, fibre and sodium content of the food. These are the key points to look for:

Energy—This is a measure of how many kilojoules (kJ) or calories we get from a food. For a healthy diet we need to eat more foods with a low energy density and combine them with smaller amounts of higher energy foods. To assess the energy density look at the kJ or Cal per 100 grams. A low energy density is less than 500 kJ per 100 g or 120 Cal per 100 g.

Fat—You want a low saturated fat content, ideally less than 20% of the total fat. This means that if the total fat content is 10 g you want saturated fat less than 2 g. Strictly speaking, a food can be labelled as low in saturated fat if it contains less than 1.5 g saturated fat/100 g.

Total carbohydrate—This is the starch plus any naturally occurring and added sugars in the food. (There's no need to look at the sugar figure separately since it's the total carbohydrate that affects your blood glucose level.) You could use this figure if you were monitoring your carbohydrate intake and to calculate the glycaemic load (GL) of your serving of the food. The GL = grams of total carbohydrate per serve × GI ÷ 100.

Fibre—Most of us don't eat enough fibre in our diet (the average intake for adults in the UK is around 12 g a day – 6 g short of the recommended 18 g a day) so it's better to look for high fibre foods. A high fibre food contains more than 6 g fibre per 100 g.

Sodium—This is a measure of the nasty part of salt in our food. Our bodies need some salt but most people consume much more than they need. Canned foods in particular tend to be high in sodium. Check the sodium content per 100 g next time you buy—a low salt food contains less than 120 mg sodium/100 g.

What to keep in your pantry

To make easy low GI choices, you'll need to stock the right foods. Here are ideas for what to keep in your pantry, refrigerator and freezer.

Asian sauces: hoi sin, oyster, soya and fish sauces are a good basic range.

Barley: one of the oldest cultivated cereals, barley is very nutritious and high in fibre. Look for products such as pearl barley to use in soups, stews and pilafs.

Black pepper: buy freshly ground pepper or grind your own peppercorns.

Bread: low GI options include granary, stoneground wholemeal, pumpernickel, sourdough, English-style muffins, flat bread and pitta bread.

Breakfast cereals: these include traditional rolled oats, natural muesli and low GI packaged breakfast cereals.

Bulgur wheat: use it to make tabbouli, or add to vegetable burgers, stuffings, soups and stews.

Canned evaporated skimmed milk: this makes an excellent substitute for cream in pasta sauces.

Canned fish: keep a good stock of canned tuna packed in spring water, and canned sardines and salmon.

Canned fruit: have a variety of canned fruit on hand, including peaches, pears, apples and nectarines—choose the brands labelled with 'no added sugar' fruit juice syrup.

Canned vegetables: sweet corn kernels and tomatoes can help to boost the vegetable content of a meal. Tomatoes, in particular, can be used freely because they are rich in anti-oxidants, as well as having a low GI.

Couscous: ready in minutes, serve with casseroles and braised dishes.

Curry pastes: a tablespoon or so makes a delicious curry base.

Dried fruit: these include sultanas, apricots, raisins, prunes and apples.

Dried herbs: oregano, basil, ground coriander, thyme and rosemary can be useful to have on stand-by in the pantry.

Honey: try to avoid the commercial honeys or honey blends, and use the Australian 'pure floral' honeys. These varieties have a much lower GI naturally.

Jam: a dollop of good-quality jam (with no added sugar) on toast contains fewer calories than butter or margarine.

Mustard: seeded or wholegrain mustard is useful as a sandwich spread, and in salad dressings and sauces.

Noodles: many Asian noodles such as Hokkien, udon and rice vermicelli have low to intermediate GI values because of their dense texture, whether they are made from wheat or rice flour.

Nuts: try a handful of nuts (about 30 g/1 oz) every other day.

Oils: try olive oil for general use; some extra-virgin olive oil for salad dressings, marinades and dishes that benefit from its flavour; and sesame oil for Asian-style stir-fries. Rapeseed or olive oil cooking sprays are handy too.

Pasta: a great source of carbohydrates and B vitamins.

Pulses: stock a variety of pulses (dried or canned), including lentils, split peas and beans. There are many bean varieties, including cannellini, butter, borlotti, kidney and soya beans.

Quinoa: this wholegrain cooks in about 10–15 minutes and has a slightly chewy texture. It can be used as a substitute for rice, couscous or bulgur wheat. It is very important to rinse the grains thoroughly before cooking.

Rice: Basmati, Doongara or Japanese koshihikari varieties are good choices because they have a lower GI than, for example, jasmine rice.

Rolled oats: besides their use in porridge, oats can be added to cakes, biscuits, breads and desserts.

Sea salt: use in moderation.

Spices: most spices, including ground cumin, turmeric, cinnamon, paprika and nutmeg, should be bought in small quantities because they lose pungency with age and incorrect storage.

Stock: make your own stock or buy ready-made products, which are available in long-life cartons in the supermarket. To keep the sodium content down with ready-made stocks, look out for a low salt option.

Tomato paste: use in soups, sauces and casseroles.

Vinegar: white wine or red wine vinegar and balsamic vinegar are excellent in vinaigrette dressings in salads.

What to keep in your refrigerator

Bacon: bacon is a valuable ingredient in many dishes because of the flavour it offers. You can make a little bacon go a long way by trimming off all fat and chopping it finely. Lean ham is often a more economical and leaner way to go.

Bottled vegetables: sun-dried tomatoes, olives and char-grilled eggplant and capsicum are handy to keep as flavoursome additions to pastas and sandwiches.

Capers, olives and anchovies: these can be bought in jars and kept in the refrigerator once opened. They are a tasty (but salty) addition to pasta dishes, salads and pizzas.

Cheese: any reduced fat cheese is great to keep handy in the fridge. A block of Parmesan is indispensable and will keep for up to a month. Reduced fat cottage and ricotta cheeses have a short life so are best bought as needed, and they can be a good alternative to butter or margarine in a sandwich.

Condiments: keep jars of minced garlic, chilli or ginger in the refrigerator to spice up your cooking in an instant.

Eggs: to enhance your intake of omega-3 fats, we suggest using omega-3-enriched eggs. Although the yolk is high in cholesterol, the fat in eggs is predominantly mono-unsaturated, and therefore considered a 'good fat'.

Fish: try a variety of fresh fish.

Fresh herbs: these are available in most supermarkets and there really is no substitute for the flavour they impart. For variety, try parsley, basil, mint, chives and coriander.

Fresh fruit: almost all fruit make an excellent low GI snack. When in season, try fruit such as apples, oranges, pears, grapes, grapefruit, peaches, apricots, strawberries and mangoes.

Meat: lean varieties are better—try lean beef, lamb fillets, pork fillets, chicken (breast or drumsticks) and minced beef.

Milk: skimmed or semi-skimmed milk is best, or try low fat calcium-enriched soya milk.

Vegetables: keep a variety of seasonal vegetables on hand such as spinach, broccoli, cauliflower, Asian greens, asparagus, courgette and mushrooms. Red pepper, spring onions and sprouts (mung bean and snowpea sprouts) are great to bulk up a salad. Sweet corn, sweet potato and yam are essential to your low GI food store.

Yoghurt: low fat natural yoghurt provides the most calcium for the fewest calories. Have vanilla or fruit versions as a dessert, or use natural yoghurt as a condiment in savoury dishes.

What to keep in your freezer

Frozen berries: berries can make any dessert special, and by using frozen ones it means you don't have to wait until berry season in order to indulge. Try berries such as blueberries, raspberries and strawberries.

Frozen yoghurt: this is a fantastic substitute for ice-cream and some products even have a similar creamy texture, but with much less fat.

Frozen vegetables: keep packets of peas, beans, corn, spinach or mixed vegetables in the freezer—these are handy to add to a quick meal.

Ice-cream: reduced or low fat ice-cream is ideal for a quick dessert, served with fresh fruit.

How we calculate the GI

As we explained earlier, the GI is simply a ranking of the carbohydrate in foods depending on their immediate effect on blood glucose levels. To make an absolutely fair comparison, all foods are tested following an internationally standardised method. The higher the GI the higher the blood glucose levels after consumption.

- A high GI value is 70 or more
- A medium GI value is 56 to 69 inclusive
- A low GI value is 55 or less

The GI rating of a food must be tested physiologically and only a few centres around the world currently provide a legitimate testing service.

Testing the GI of a food requires a group of eight to ten subjects and knowledge of the food's carbohydrate content. After an overnight fast, each subject consumes a portion of the test food containing a specified amount of carbohydrate (usually 50 grams, but sometimes 25 or even 15 grams). Fingerprick blood samples are taken at 15- to 30-minute intervals over the next two hours. During this time, blood glucose levels rise and fall back to baseline levels. The full extent of glycaemia (rise in blood glucose) is assessed by measuring the area under the curve using a computer algorithm. For example, our subject, Lisa, eats a 50-gram carbohydrate portion of barley. Her area under the curve was found to be 60 units.

On three other occasions our subjects must consume the reference food (the same amount of carbohydrate given as pure glucose) to determine their average response to the reference food. Our subject Lisa was found to have an average area of 180 units. Each subject's area under the curve to the test food is then expressed as a percentage of their average after the reference food. Lisa's value is $(60/180) \times 100 = 30$. Hence the GI of barley in Lisa's case is 30. There will be some variation between subjects but if we were to test them again and again, all subjects will tend to move towards the average of the whole group.

Is there an easier way to test the GI of a food? No! The GI is *defined* by its standardised method of testing in human subjects (*in vivo* testing). You may hear about *in vitro* (test tube) methods but these are simple short-cut methods that may or may not reflect the true GI of a food. *In vitro* methods may guide food manufacturers during re-formulation of their product, but only *in vivo* testing can give us a GI value.

In the following tables we have also included some foods that contain very little carbohydrate or none at all because so many people ask us for their GI. Many vegetables such as avocado and broccoli, and protein-rich foods such as eggs, cheese, chicken and tuna are among the low or no carbohydrate category. We show this as ★. Most alcoholic beverages are also low in carbohydrate.

Let's talk glycaemic load (GL)

In addition to the GI values, the tables in this book include the GL (glycaemic load) of normal-sized portions of the food on your plate. Glycaemic load is the product of GI and the amount of carbohydrate in a serving of food. You can think about GL as the amount of carbohydrate 'adjusted' for its GI. This means that you can choose foods with either a low GI and/or a low GL.

When we eat a meal containing carbohydrate, our blood glucose rises and falls. The extent to which it rises and remains high is critically important to health and depends on two things: the amount of carbohydrate in the meal and the nature of that carbohydrate (its GI value). Both are equally important determinants of changes in blood glucose levels.

Researchers at Harvard University came up with a way of combining and describing these two factors with the term 'glycaemic load'. The glycaemic load helps us predict what the effect of a particular carbohydrate food will be on our blood glucose level after consuming that food. The glycaemic load is greatest for high GI foods containing the most carbohydrate (such as rice or bread), especially when eaten in large quantities.

Don't get carried away with glycaemic load. The glycaemic load doesn't distinguish 'slow carbs' from 'low carbs'. It is much better to make food choices based on the GI rather than the GL because you want to see at least moderate amounts of carbohydrates in your meal. If you choose only on the basis of glycaemic load, you could easily find yourself eating a lot of unwanted fat and excess protein. Low GI carbohydrates give you much more than just control of blood glucose—you'll feel fuller for longer thanks to prolonged absorption and you'll reduce your insulin levels at the same time.

The glycaemic load is calculated simply by multiplying the GI value of a food by the amount of carbohydrate per serving and dividing by 100.

Glycaemic load (GL) =
(GI value × carbohydrate per serving) ÷ 100

For example, an apple has a GI value of 40 and contains 15 grams of carbohydrate per serving. Its GL is:

$$(40 \times 15) \div 100 = 6.$$

A potato has a GI value of 90 and 20 grams of carbohydrate per serving. It has a GL of:

$$(90 \times 20) \div 100 = 18.$$

This is not to say that the glycaemic response will be exactly three times higher for a potato compared with an apple, but the total metabolic effect, including overall insulin demand, might be three times higher.

Don't use the GL values in isolation!

If you use GL values alone, you might find yourself eating a diet with *very little carbohydrate* and, as mentioned above, a whole heap of fat, especially saturated fat, and excessive amounts of protein! GL does not distinguish between '**low** carb' and '**slow** carb'.

So what should you do?

- *Use the GI to compare foods of a similar nature (breads with breads); **the low GI varieties will have the lower GL values**.*
- *Use the GL when comparing foods with a high GI but low carbohydrate content per serving.*

Remember that the GL values listed in the following tables are for the specified nominal portion size. If you eat more (or less) you will need to calculate another GL value.

Low GL = 10 or less
Medium GL = 11–19
High GL = 20 or more

Look for the GI on the foods you buy

A GI symbol on the packet tells you that a food has been glycaemic index tested. Unfortunately, not all claims are reliable.

The GI Symbol Programme

This symbol on foods is your guarantee that the product meets the GI Symbol Programme's strict nutritional criteria. Whether high, medium or low GI, you can be assured that these foods are healthier choices within their food group and will make a nutritious contribution to your diet. *

The GI Symbol Programme is an international programme that was established by the University of Sydney, Diabetes Australia and the Juvenile Diabetes Research Foundation – organisations whose expertise in GI is recognised around the world. The logo is a trademark of the University of Sydney in Australia and in other countries including the UK. A food product carrying this logo is nutritious and has been tested for its GI in an accredited laboratory. For more information, visit www.gisymbol.com

Some UK supermarket chains are progressively testing and labelling their foods.

- **Tesco** have had a number of foods glycaemic index tested by Oxford Brookes University and these foods have been included in this book and are available on their website (www.tesco.com).
- **Sainsbury's** are launching GI labelling progressively across a range of products that meet strict nutritional criteria and backing this with a comprehensive guide to GI on their website (www.sainsburys.co. uk). The products have been tested by Hammersmith Hospital Food Research Company.

We will include new foods in our comprehensive tables as soon as they become available and we have had an opportunity to evaluate them.

Note: The GI values in this book are correct at the time of publication. However, the formulation of commercial foods can change and the GI may change as well.

A to Z
GI Values

Consult these tables when you want to locate the GI value of a popular food quickly. Here foods are listed alphabetically—both on an individual basis and within their specific food category. For example, you will find apple juice under both 'Apple juice' and 'Fruit and vegetable juice'. Food category entries include:

Bakery products	Honey
Beverages	Ice-cream
Biscuits	Meat
Bread	Milk
Breakfast cereal bars	Muffins
Breakfast cereals	Noodles
Cakes	Nuts
Cereal grains	Pasta
Chocolate	Pizza
Crackers and crispbreads	Potatoes
Dairy products	Pre-packed meals
Fruit	Pulses
Fruit and vegetable juices	Rice

Seafood

Snack foods

Soft drinks

Soups

Soya milk

Soya products

Sports drinks

Spreads

Tesco breads

Tesco breakfast cereals

Vegetables

White bread

Wholemeal bread

Yoghurt

Key

★ Means that a food has such a low carbohydrate content that the GI cannot be measured.
See pages 26–27 for more details on measuring a food's GI.

■ Means that a food may be high in saturated fat. As we have mentioned previously, the GI should not be used in isolation, but the overall nutritional value of the food needs to be considered.

Ⓖ Means that a food has been accurately tested for its GI and meets strict nutritional criteria. You can be assured that these foods are healthier choices within their food group.

FOOD	GI	NOMINAL SERVE SIZE	AVAILABLE CARB PER SERVE	GL PER SERVE
Alfalfa sprouts	★	6 g	0	0
All-Bran®, breakfast cereal, Kellogg's®	34	30 g	15	4
Angel food cake, plain	67■	50 g	29	19
Apple, dried	29	60 g	34	10
Apple, fresh	38	120 g	15	6
Apple juice, Granny Smith, unsweetened	44	200 ml	24	10
Apple juice, no added sugar	40	250 ml	28	11
Apple muffin, home-made	46■	60 g	29	13
Apricots, canned in light syrup	64	120 g	19	12
Apricots, dried, ready to eat	31	60 g	22	7
Apricots, dried, ready to eat, bite size	32	60 g	22	7
Apricots, fresh	57	168 g	13	7
Arborio, risotto rice, white, boiled	69	150 g	43	29
Artichokes, globe, fresh or canned in brine	★	80 g	0	0
Arugula	★	30 g	0	0
Asparagus	★	100 g	0	0
Aubergine	★	100 g	0	0
Avocado	★	120 g	0	0
Bacon	★	50 g	0	0
Bagel, white	72	70 g	35	25

FOOD	GI	NOMINAL SERVE SIZE	AVAILABLE CARB PER SERVE	GL PER SERVE
Baked beans, canned in tomato sauce	49	150 g	17	8
BAKERY PRODUCTS				
Bagel, white	72	70 g	35	25
Croissant, plain	67■	57 g	26	17
Crumpet, white	69	50 g	19	13
Scones, plain, made from packet mix	92	25 g	9	8
Banana cake, home-made	51■	80 g	38	18
Banana, raw	52	120 g	26	13
Banana smoothie, low fat	30	250 ml	26	8
Barley, pearled, boiled	25	150 g	32	8
Basmati rice, boiled, Tesco Value	52	75 g	40	21
Basmati rice, Indian, boiled	69	75 g	57	39
Basmati rice, Indian, easy cook, boiled	67	75 g	60	40
Basmati rice, organic, boiled	57	75 g	57	33
Bean curd, tofu, plain, unsweetened	★	100 g	0	0
Bean sprouts, raw	★	14 g	0	0
Bean thread noodles, dried, boiled	33	180 g	45	12
Beef	★■	120 g	0	0
Beef and ale casserole, Tesco Finest	53	300 g	15	8
Beetroot, canned	64	80 g	7	5

★ little or no carbs ■ high in saturated fat

B

FOOD	GI	NOMINAL SERVE SIZE	AVAILABLE CARB PER SERVE	GL PER SERVE
BEVERAGES				
Probiotic drink, cranberry	56	100 ml	12	7
Probiotic drink, orange	30	100 ml	13	4
Probiotic drink, original	34	100 ml	12	4
Probiotic drink, pink grapefruit	60	100 ml	13	8
Probiotic yoghurt, prune	44	170 ml	24	11
Probiotic yoghurt, raspberry	45	170 ml	24	11
Probiotic yoghurt, strawberry	52	170 ml	24	13
BISCUITS				
Digestive biscuits, plain	59■	25 g	16	10
Oatcakes	57■	25 g	15	8
Rich Tea® biscuits	55■	25 g	19	10
Shortbread, plain	64■	25 g	16	10
Wafer biscuits, vanilla, plain	77■	25 g	18	14
Black-eyed beans, soaked, boiled	42	150 g	29	12
Black beans, boiled	30	150 g	25	5
Black bean soup, canned	64	250 ml	27	17
Black rye bread	76	30 g	13	10
Blueberry muffin, commercially made	59■	57 g	29	17
Bok choy	★	100 g	0	0
Borlotti beans, canned, drained	41	75 g	12	5
Bran Flakes™, breakfast cereal, Kellogg's®	74	30 g	18	13

FOOD	GI	NOMINAL SERVE SIZE	AVAILABLE CARB PER SERVE	GL PER SERVE
Bran muffin, commercially made	60■	57 g	24	15
Brawn	★■	75 g	0	0
BREAD				
Black rye bread	76	30 g	13	10
Crusty malted wheat bread, Tesco Finest	52	30 g	13	7
Dark rye bread	86	30 g	14	12
Fruit & Muesli loaf, Bürgen®	51	45 g	29	15
Fruit and cinnamon bread, Tesco Finest	71	37 g	20	14
Fruit loaf, sliced	57	30 g	16	9
Fruit loaf, Tesco Value	90	30 g	18	16
Fruit loaf, thick sliced	47	30 g	15	7
Hamburger bun, white	61	30 g	15	9
Light rye bread	68	30 g	14	10
Malt loaf, organic	59	35 g	24	13
Melba toast, plain	70	30 g	23	16
Multi-grain batch bread	62	50 g	24	15
Multigrain sandwich bread	65	30 g	28	18
Oatmeal batch bread	62	50 g	25	16
Pitta bread, white	57	30 g	17	10
Pitta bread, white, mini	68	30 g	15	10
Pitta bread, white, Tesco Value	69	60 g	31	21
Pitta bread, wholemeal	56	60 g	28	16

B

★ little or no carbs ■ high in saturated fat

B

FOOD	GI	NOMINAL SERVE SIZE	AVAILABLE CARB PER SERVE	GL PER SERVE
Pumpernickel bread	50	30 g	10	5
Roll (bread), white	73	30 g	16	12
Rye bread, wholemeal	51	40 g	13	7
Sourdough bread, organic, stoneground, wholemeal	59	32 g	12	7
Sourdough rye bread	48	30 g	12	6
Sourdough wheat bread	54	30 g	14	8
Soya and Linseed, Bürgen®	55	70 g	24	13
Vogel's Honey and Oat Bran bread	49	40 g	13	7
White bread, regular, sliced	71	30 g	14	10
BREAKFAST CEREAL BARS				
Crunchy Nut Corn Flakes Bar, Kellogg's®	72	30 g	26	19
BREAKFAST CEREALS				
All-Bran®, Kellogg's®	34	30 g	15	5
Bran Flakes, Kellogg's®	74	30 g	18	13
Branflakes, Tesco Healthy Living	50	30 g	20	10
Coco Pops®, Kellogg's®	77	30 g	26	20
Corn Flakes®, Kellogg's®	77	30 g	25	20
Crunchy Nut Corn Flakes, Kellogg's®	72	30 g	24	17
Frosties®, Kellogg's®	55	30 g	26	15
Fruit and fibre breakfast cereal	67	30 g	21	14
Fruit and fibre cereal, Tesco Value	68	40 g	26	18

FOOD	GI	NOMINAL SERVE SIZE	AVAILABLE CARB PER SERVE	GL PER SERVE
Hi fibre bran cereal	43	30 g	12	5
Muesli, fruit	67	50 g	34	23
Muesli, fruit and nut	59	50 g	30	18
Muesli, Tesco Healthy Eating	86	50 g	36	31
Muesli, Tesco Value	64	50 g	31	20
Muesli, wholewheat	56	50 g	30	17
Oat bran, raw, unprocessed	55	10 g	5	3
Oats, rolled, raw	59	50 g	31	18
Porridge, instant, made with water	82	30 g	26	17
Porridge oats, organic	63	50 g	29	18
Porridge oats, Scottish	63	50 g	31	20
Porridge oats, Tesco Value	63	50 g	30	19
Porridge, regular, made from oats with water	58	250 g	21	11
Puffed Wheat	80	30 g	21	17
Rice Krispies®, Kellogg's®	82	30 g	26	22
Semolina, cooked	55	150 g	11	6
Shredded Wheat	75	30 g	20	15
Special K®, regular, Kellogg's®	56	30 g	21	11
Sultana bran, Tesco Healthy Living	90	30 g	17	16
Sultana Bran™, Kellogg's®	73	30 g	19	14
Broad beans	79	80 g	11	9
Broccoli	★	60 g	0	0
Brussels sprouts	★	100 g	0	0

★ little or no carbs ■ high in saturated fat

B

C

FOOD	GI	NOMINAL SERVE SIZE	AVAILABLE CARB PER SERVE	GL PER SERVE
Buckwheat, boiled	54	150 g	30	16
Buckwheat, puffed	65	14 g	12	8
Bulgur, cracked wheat, ready to eat	48	150 g	26	12
Bun, hamburger, white	61	30 g	15	9
Butter beans, canned, drained	36	75 g	12	4
Butter beans, dried, soaked overnight, boiled	26	150 g	75	19
Cabbage	★	70 g	0	0
CAKES				
Angel food cake, plain	67■	50 g	29	19
Banana cake, home-made	51■	80 g	38	18
Chocolate cake, made from packet mix with icing	38■	110 g	52	20
Cupcake, strawberry-iced	73■	38 g	26	19
Pound cake, plain	54■	50 g	23	12
Sponge cake, plain, unfilled	46■	63 g	36	17
Vanilla cake made from packet mix with vanilla frosting	42■	111 g	58	24
Calamari rings, squid, not battered or crumbed	★	70 g	0	0
Cannellini beans	31	85 g	12	4
Cannelloni, spinach and ricotta	15	400 g	72	11
Cantaloupe	67	120 g	6	4
Carrot juice, freshly made	43	250 ml	23	10

FOOD	GI	NOMINAL SERVE SIZE	AVAILABLE CARB PER SERVE	GL PER SERVE
Carrots, peeled, boiled	41	80 g	5	2
Cashew nut halves	27	50 g	10	3
Cashew nuts	25	50 g	12	3
Cashew nuts, organic, roasted and salted	25	50 g	12	3
Cashew nuts, roasted and salted	27	50 g	10	3
Cauliflower	★	60 g	0	0
Celery	★	40 g	0	0
CEREAL GRAINS				
Barley, pearled, boiled	25	150 g	32	8
Buckwheat, boiled	54	150 g	30	16
Buckwheat, puffed	65	14 g	12	8
Bulgur, cracked wheat, ready to eat	48	150 g	26	12
Cornmeal (polenta), boiled	68	150 g	13	9
Couscous, boiled 5 mins	65	150 g	33	21
Polenta, boiled	68	150 g	13	9
Quinoa, organic, boiled	53	100 g	17	9
Rye, grain	34	50 g	38	13
Semolina, cooked	55	150 g	11	6
Cheese	★■	120 g	0	0
Cheese tortellini, cooked	50■	180 g	21	10
Cherries, dark, raw	63	120 g	12	3
Chicken	★	110 g	0	0

★ little or no carbs ■ high in saturated fat 43

Chicken korma and peshwari rice, pre-packed

FOOD	GI	NOMINAL SERVE SIZE	AVAILABLE CARB PER SERVE	GL PER SERVE
Chicken korma and peshwari rice, pre-packed, Tesco Finest	44	550 g	88	39
Chicken korma and rice, pre-packed, Tesco Healthy Living	45	450 g	72	32
Chicken nuggets, frozen, reheated in microwave 5 mins	46■	100 g	16	7
Chicken, sweet and sour with noodles (Serves One)	41	475 g	82	33
Chicken, tandoori, masala and rice, pre-packed, Tesco Finest	45	550 g	112	50
Chicken tikka masala and rice, pre-packed, Tesco Healthy Living	34	550 g	111	38
Chickpeas, canned in brine	40	150 g	22	9
Chickpeas, dried, boiled	28	150 g	24	7
Chilli beef noodles, Tesco Finest	42	450 g	68	29
Chillies, fresh or dried	★	20 g	0	0
Chives, fresh	★	4 g	0	0
CHOCOLATE				
Chocolate cake, made from packet mix with icing	38■	110 g	52	20
Chocolate, dark, plain	41■	30 g	19	8
Chocolate, milk, plain, Cadbury's®	49■	30 g	17	8
Chocolate, white, plain, Nestlé®	44■	50 g	29	13
M&M's®, peanut	33■	30 g	17	6
Mars Bar®, regular	62■	60 g	40	25

★ little or no carbs ■ high in saturated fat

Chocolate—Milky Bar®, plain white chocolate, Nestlé

FOOD	GI	NOMINAL SERVE SIZE	AVAILABLE CARB PER SERVE	GL PER SERVE
Milky Bar®, plain white chocolate, Nestlé®	44■	50 g	29	13
Twix® bar	44■	60 g	39	17
Chow mein, chicken (Serves One)	47	475 g	60	28
Chow mein, chicken, Tesco Healthy Living	55	450 g	34	19
Coca-Cola®, soft drink	53	250 ml	26	14
Coco Pops®, breakfast cereal, Kellogg's®	77	30 g	26	20
Condensed milk, sweetened, full fat	61■	50 ml	28	17
Consommé, clear, chicken or vegetable	★	205 ml	2	0
Corn Flakes, breakfast cereal, Kellogg's®	77	30 g	25	20
Cornmeal (polenta), boiled	68	150 g	13	9
Corn, sweet, on the cob, boiled	48	80 g	16	8
Corn, sweet, whole kernel, canned, drained	46	80 g	14	7
Cottage pie, pre-packed	65	500 g	56	36
Courgette	★	100 g	0	0
Couscous, boiled 5 mins	65	150 g	33	21

CRACKERS AND CRISPBREADS

FOOD	GI	NOMINAL SERVE SIZE	AVAILABLE CARB PER SERVE	GL PER SERVE
Melba toast, plain	70	30 g	23	16
Rice cakes, puffed, white	82	25 g	21	17
Water crackers, plain	78	25 g	18	14

★ little or no carbs ■ high in saturated fat   45

Cranberries, dried, sweetened

FOOD	GI	NOMINAL SERVE SIZE	AVAILABLE CARB PER SERVE	GL PER SERVE
Cranberries, dried, sweetened	64	40 g	29	19
Cranberry Juice Cocktail, Ocean Spray	52	250 ml	31	16
Croissant, plain	67■	57 g	26	17
Crumpet, white	69	50 g	19	13
Crunchy Nut Corn Flakes Bar, Kellogg's®	72	30 g	26	19
Cucumber	★	45 g	0	0
Cumberland fish pie, pre-packed	40	250 g	26	10
Cumberland pie, pre-packed	29	500 g	62	18
Cupcake, strawberry-iced	73■	38 g	26	19
Custard apple, fresh, flesh only	54	120 g	19	10
Custard, home-made from milk, wheat starch and sugar	43■	100 ml	17	7
Custard, vanilla, reduced fat	37	100 ml	15	6

DAIRY PRODUCTS

FOOD	GI	NOMINAL SERVE SIZE	AVAILABLE CARB PER SERVE	GL PER SERVE
Cheese	★■	120 g	0	0
Custard, home-made from milk, wheat starch and sugar	43■	100 ml	17	7
Vanilla custard, reduced fat	37	100 ml	15	6
Dark rye bread	86	30 g	14	12
Dates, Arabic, dried, vacuum-packed	39	55 g	41	16
Dates, dried	103	60 g	40	42

FOOD	GI	NOMINAL SERVE SIZE	AVAILABLE CARB PER SERVE	GL PER SERVE
Desiree potato, peeled, boiled 35 mins	101	150 g	17	17
Diet jelly, made from crystals with water	★	125 g	0	0
Diet soft drinks	★	250 ml	0	0
Digestive biscuits, plain	59■	25 g	16	10
Dried apple	29	60 g	34	10
Duck	★■	140 g	0	0
Eggs	★■	120 g	0	0
Endive	★	30 g	0	0
Fajitas, chicken	42	275 g	39	17
Fanta®, orange soft drink	68	250 ml	34	23
Fat-free yoghurts, various flavours	40	200g	31	12
Fennel	★	90 g	0	0
Fettuccine, egg, cooked	40	180 g	46	18
Figs, dried, tenderised	61	60 g	26	16
Fish	★	120 g	0	0
Fish fingers	38■	100 g	19	7
Four bean mix, canned, drained	37	75 g	12	5
French fries, frozen, reheated in microwave	75■	150 g	29	22
Frosties®, breakfast cereal, Kellogg's®	55	30 g	26	15
Fructose, pure	19	10 g	10	2

D

E

F

Fruit & Muesli loaf, Bürgen

FOOD	GI	NOMINAL SERVE SIZE	AVAILABLE CARB PER SERVE	GL PER SERVE
Fruit & Muesli loaf, Bürgen®	51	45 g	29	15
Fruit and fibre breakfast cereal	67	30 g	21	14
Fruit and nut mix, Tesco Finest	15	50 g	24	3
Fruit and nut mix, tropical, Tesco Finest	49	50 g	28	14
FRUIT AND VEGETABLE JUICE				
Apple juice, no added sugar	40	250 ml	28	11
Carrot juice, freshly made	43	250 ml	23	10
Cranberry Juice Cocktail, Ocean Spray	52	250 ml	31	16
Granny Smith apple juice, unsweetened	44	200 ml	24	10
Grapefruit juice, unsweetened	48	250 ml	22	9
Orange juice, unsweetened	50	250 ml	18	9
Pineapple juice, unsweetened	46	250 ml	34	16
Tomato juice, no added sugar	38	250 ml	9	4
FRUIT, CANNED				
Apricots in light syrup	64	120 g	19	12
Lychees in syrup, drained	79	120 g	20	16
Peaches in heavy syrup	58	120 g	15	9
Peaches in light syrup	57	120 g	18	9
Peaches in natural juice	45	120 g	11	4
Pear halves in natural juice	44	120 g	13	5
Pear halves in reduced-sugar syrup	25	120 g	14	4

★ little or no carbs ■ high in saturated fat

FOOD	GI	NOMINAL SERVE SIZE	AVAILABLE CARB PER SERVE	GL PER SERVE
FRUIT, DRIED				
Apple	29	60 g	34	10
Apricots, dried, ready to eat	31	60 g	22	7
Apricots, dried, ready to eat, bite size	32	60 g	22	7
Cranberries, sweetened	64	40 g	29	19
Dates, Arabic, vacuum-packed	39	55 g	41	16
Dates	103	60 g	40	42
Figs, tenderised	61	60 g	26	16
Mixed fruit, dried, Tesco Value	60	60 g	41	6
Peaches, dried, ready to eat	35	60 g	22	8
Pears, dried, ready to eat	43	60 g	27	12
Prunes, pitted	29	60 g	33	10
Raisins	64	60 g	44	28
Sultanas	58	60 g	42	24
Sultanas, Tesco Value	56	60 g	42	24
FRUIT, FRESH				
Apple	38	120 g	15	6
Apricots	57	168 g	13	7
Avocado	★	120 g	0	0
Banana	52	120 g	26	13
Cantaloupe	67	120 g	6	4
Cherries, dark	63	120 g	12	3
Custard apple, flesh only	54	120 g	19	10

★ little or no carbs   ■ high in saturated fat

F

FOOD	GI	NOMINAL SERVE SIZE	AVAILABLE CARB PER SERVE	GL PER SERVE
Grapefruit	25	120 g	11	3
Grapes	53	120 g	18	8
Kiwi fruit	53	120 g	12	6
Lemon	★	40 g	0	0
Lime	★	40 g	0	0
Mango	51	120 g	17	8
Orange	42	120 g	11	5
Paw paw	56	120 g	8	5
Peach	42	120 g	11	5
Pear	38	120 g	11	4
Pineapple	59	120 g	10	6
Plum	39	120 g	12	5
Raspberries	★	65 g	0	0
Rhubarb	★	125 g	0	0
Strawberries	40	120 g	3	1
Watermelon	76	120 g	6	4
Fruit loaf, sliced	57	30 g	16	9
Fusilli pasta twists, dry pasta, boiled	54	50 g	36	20
Fusilli pasta twists, tricolour, dry pasta, boiled	51	50 g	34	17
Fusilli pasta twists, wholewheat, dry pasta, boiled	55	50 g	31	17
G Garlic	★	5 g	0	0

★ little or no carbs ■ high in saturated fat

FOOD	GI	NOMINAL SERVE SIZE	AVAILABLE CARB PER SERVE	GL PER SERVE
Ginger	★	10 g	0	0
Glucose tablets	100	10 g	10	10
Glutinous rice, white, cooked in rice cooker	98	150 g	32	31
Gnocchi, cooked	68	180 g	48	33
Golden syrup	63	20 g	17	11
Granny Smith apple juice, unsweetened	44	200 ml	24	10
Grapefruit, fresh	25	120 g	11	3
Grapefruit juice, unsweetened	48	250 ml	22	9
Grapes, fresh	53	120 g	18	8
Green beans	★	70 g	0	0
Green pea soup, canned	66	250 ml	41	27
Hamburger bun, white	61	30 g	15	9
Ham, leg or shoulder	★■	24 g	0	0
Haricot beans, cooked, canned	38	150 g	31	12
Haricot beans, dried, boiled	33	150 g	31	10
Heinz® Baked Beans in tomato sauce, canned	49	150 g	17	8
Herbs, fresh or dried	★	2 g	0	0
Hi fibre bran cereal	43	30 g	12	5
Hommous, regular	6	30 g	5	1
Honey and Oat Bran bread, Vogel's	49	40g	13	7

G

H

★ little or no carbs ■ high in saturated fat

FOOD	GI	NOMINAL SERVE SIZE	AVAILABLE CARB PER SERVE	GL PER SERVE
HONEY				
Honey, pure floral	35	25 g	18	6
Honey, various (averaged)	55	25 g	18	10
Ice-cream, vanilla, full fat	38■	50 g	9	3
ICE-CREAM				
Vanilla ice-cream, full fat	38■	50 g	9	3
Instant mashed potato	85	150 g	20	17
Instant noodles, 99% fat free	67	75 g	51	34
Instant noodles, regular	54■	180 g	23	10
Instant rice, white, cooked 6 mins	87	150 g	42	36
Isostar® sports drink	70	250 ml	18	13
Jasmine rice, white, long-grain, cooked in rice cooker	109	150 g	42	46
Jelly beans	78	30 g	28	22
Jelly, diet, made from crystals with water	★	125 g	0	0
Kidney beans, dark red, canned, drained	43	150 g	25	7
Kidney beans, red, canned, drained	36	150 g	17	9
Kidney beans, red, dried, soaked overnight, boiled	51	150 g	60	31
Kiwi fruit, fresh	53	120 g	12	6
Lamb	★	120 g	0	0

FOOD	GI	NOMINAL SERVE SIZE	AVAILABLE CARB PER SERVE	GL PER SERVE
Lamb moussaka, pre-packed, Tesco Finest	35	330 g	30	11
Lasagne	25	400 g	40	10
Lasagne, beef, frozen	47	400 g	47	22
Lasagne, egg, dry pasta, boiled	53	50 g	33	18
Lasagne, egg, verdi, dry pasta, boiled	52	50 g	35	18
Lasagne, meat, chilled, Tesco Healthy Living	28	340 g	43	12
Lasagne sheets, dry pasta, boiled, Tesco Value	55	50 g	36	20
Lasagne, Tesco Finest	34	300 g	31	10
Lasagne, vegetarian	20	430 g	69	14
Leeks	★	80 g	0	0
Lemon	★	40 g	0	0
Lentil soup, canned	44	250 ml	21	9
Lentils, red, split, boiled	21	150 g	77	16
Lettuce	★	50 g	0	0
Licorice, soft	78	60 g	42	33
Light rye bread	68	30 g	14	10
Lima beans, baby, frozen, reheated	32	150 g	30	10
Lime	★	40 g	0	0
Linguine pasta, thick, durum wheat, boiled	46	180 g	48	22
Linguine pasta, thin, durum wheat, boiled	52	180 g	45	23

★ little or no carbs ■ high in saturated fat

L

FOOD	GI	NOMINAL SERVE SIZE	AVAILABLE CARB PER SERVE	GL PER SERVE
Linseed and Soya Loaf, bread	55	70 g	24	13
Liver sausage	★■	30 g	0	0
Low fat soya milk, calcium-fortified	44	250 ml	17	8
Lucozade®, original, sparkling glucose drink	95	250 ml	42	40
Lychees, canned, in syrup, drained	79	120 g	20	16

M

FOOD	GI	NOMINAL SERVE SIZE	AVAILABLE CARB PER SERVE	GL PER SERVE
M&M's®, peanut	33■	30 g	17	6
Macaroni, white, plain, boiled	47	180 g	48	23
Malt loaf, organic	59	35 g	24	13
Mango, fresh	51	120 g	17	8
Maple syrup, pure, Canadian	54	24 g	18	10
Mars Bar®, regular	62■	60 g	40	25
Marshmallows, plain, pink and white	62	25 g	20	12
MEAT				
Bacon	★	50 g	0	0
Beef	★■	120 g	0	0
Brawn	★■	75 g	0	0
Chicken	★	110 g	0	0
Duck	★■	140 g	0	0
Ham, leg or shoulder	★■	24 g	0	0
Lamb	★	120 g	0	0
Liver sausage	★■	30 g	0	0
Pork	★■	120 g	0	0

FOOD	GI	NOMINAL SERVE SIZE	AVAILABLE CARB PER SERVE	GL PER SERVE
Salami	★■	120 g	0	0
Sausages, fried	28■	100 g	3	1
Steak, any cut	★■	120 g	0	0
Turkey	★■	140 g	0	0
Veal	★	120 g	0	0
Melba toast, plain	70	30 g	23	16
MILK				
Condensed milk, sweetened, full fat	61■	50 ml	28	17
Semi-skimmed, low fat (1.4%)	32	250 ml	12	4
Semi-skimmed, pasteurised, British, Dairycrest	25	250 ml	13	3
Semi-skimmed, pasteurised, organic, Arla	34	250 ml	13	4
Skimmed, low fat (0.1%)	32	250 ml	12	4
Skimmed, pasteurised, British, Dairycrest	48	250 ml	13	6
Soya, calcium-enriched	36	250 ml	18	6
Standardised homogenised, pasteurised, British, Dairycrest	46	250 ml	12	5
Whole, pasteurised, fresh, organic, Arla	34	250 ml	12	4
Milky Bar®, plain white chocolate, Nestlé®	44■	50 g	29	13
Minestrone soup, traditional, canned	39	250 ml	18	7

★ little or no carbs ■ high in saturated fat   55

FOOD	GI	NOMINAL SERVE SIZE	AVAILABLE CARB PER SERVE	GL PER SERVE
Mixed fruit, dried, Tesco Value	60	60 g	41	6
Muesli bar, chewy, with choc chips or fruit	54■	31 g	21	12
Muesli bar, crunchy, with dried fruit	61	30 g	21	13
Muesli, fruit	67	50 g	34	23
Muesli, fruit and nut	59	50 g	30	18
Muesli, wholewheat	56	50 g	30	17
MUFFINS				
Apple muffin, home-made	46■	60 g	29	13
Blueberry muffin, commercially made	59■	57 g	29	17
Bran muffin, commercially made	60■	57 g	24	15
Multi-grain batch bread	62	50 g	24	15
Multigrain sandwich bread	65	30 g	28	18
Mung bean noodles (bean thread), dried, boiled	33	180 g	45	18
Mung beans	39	150 g	17	5
Mushrooms	★	35 g	0	0
Mushroom stroganoff with rice	26	400 g	58	15
New potato, canned, microwaved 3 mins	65	150 g	18	12
New potato, unpeeled and boiled 20 mins	78	150 g	21	13
NOODLES				
Bean thread noodles, dried, boiled	33	180 g	45	12

N

FOOD	GI	NOMINAL SERVE SIZE	AVAILABLE CARB PER SERVE	GL PER SERVE
Instant noodles, 99% fat free	67	75 g	51	34
Instant noodles, regular	54■	180 g	23	10
Mung bean noodles (bean thread), dried, boiled	33	180 g	45	18
Rice noodles, dried, boiled	61	176 g	39	24
Rice noodles, fresh, boiled	40	180 g	39	15
Rice vermicelli, dried, boiled	58	180 g	39	22
2 minute noodles (99% fat free), Maggi	71	75	51	34
2 minute noodles, regular, Maggi	54	75	51	34
Nutella®, hazelnut spread	33	20 g	12	4
NUTS				
Cashew nut halves	27	50 g	10	3
Cashew nuts	25	50 g	12	3
Cashew nuts, organic, roasted and salted	25	50 g	12	3
Cashew nuts, roasted and salted	27	50 g	10	3
Fruit and nut mix, Tesco Finest	15	50 g	24	3
Mixed nuts and raisins	21	50 g	16	3
Mixed nuts, roasted and salted	24	50 g	17	4
Peanuts, roasted, salted	14	50 g	6	1
Pecan nuts, raw	10	50 g	3	0
Tropical fruit and nut mix, Tesco Finest	49	50 g	28	14
Nuts and raisins, mixed	21	50 g	16	3

★ little or no carbs   ■ high in saturated fat

Nuts, mixed, roasted and salted

FOOD	GI	NOMINAL SERVE SIZE	AVAILABLE CARB PER SERVE	GL PER SERVE
N				
Nuts, mixed, roasted and salted	24	50 g	17	4
O				
Oat bran, unprocessed	55	10 g	5	3
Oatcakes	57■	25 g	15	8
Oatmeal batch bread	62	50 g	25	16
Oats, rolled, raw	59	50 g	31	18
Okra	★	80 g	0	0
Onions, raw, peeled	★	30 g	0	0
Orange, fresh	42	120 g	11	5
Orange juice, unsweetened	50	250 ml	18	9
Organic stoneground wholemeal sourdough bread	59	32 g	12	7
Oysters, natural, plain	★	85 g	0	0
P				
Parsnips	97	80 g	12	12
Pasta bake, tomato and mozzarella	23	340 g	48	11
PASTA				
Cannelloni, spinach and ricotta	15	400 g	72	11
Fettuccine, egg, cooked	40	180 g	46	18
Fusilli pasta twists, dry pasta, boiled	54	50 g	36	20
Fusilli pasta twists, tricolour, dry pasta, boiled	51	50 g	34	17
Fusilli pasta twists, wholewheat, dry pasta, boiled	55	50 g	31	17
Gnocchi, cooked	68	180 g	48	33

FOOD	GI	NOMINAL SERVE SIZE	AVAILABLE CARB PER SERVE	GL PER SERVE
Lasagne	25	400 g	40	10
Lasagne, egg, dry pasta, boiled	53	50 g	33	18
Lasagne, egg, verdi, dry pasta, boiled	52	50 g	35	18
Lasagne sheets, dry pasta, boiled, Tesco Value	55	50 g	36	20
Lasagne, vegetarian	20	430 g	69	14
Linguine, thick, durum wheat, boiled	46	180 g	48	22
Linguine, thin, durum wheat, boiled	52	180 g	45	23
Macaroni, white, plain, boiled	47	180 g	48	23
Pasta bake, tomato and mozzarella	23	340 g	48	11
Ravioli, meat-filled, durum wheat flour, boiled	39■	180 g	38	15
Rice pasta, brown, gluten-free, boiled	92	180 g	38	35
Rice pasta, brown, boiled	92	180 g	38	35
Spaghetti, gluten-free, rice and split pea, canned in tomato sauce	68	220 g	27	19
Spaghetti, white, durum wheat, boiled 10–15 mins	44	180 g	48	21
Spaghetti, wholemeal, boiled	42	180 g	42	16
Spirali, white, durum wheat, boiled	43	180 g	44	19
Tagliatelle, egg, dry pasta, boiled	46	50 g	33	15
Tortellini, cheese, boiled	50■	180 g	21	10
Vermicelli, white, durum wheat, boiled	35	180 g	44	16
Paw paw, fresh	56	120 g	8	5

★ little or no carbs   ■ high in saturated fat   59

Peach, fresh

FOOD	GI	NOMINAL SERVE SIZE	AVAILABLE CARB PER SERVE	GL PER SERVE
Peach, fresh	42	120 g	11	5
Peaches, canned, in heavy syrup	58	120 g	15	9
Peaches, canned, in light syrup	57	120 g	18	9
Peaches, canned, in natural juice	45	120 g	11	4
Peaches, dried, ready to eat	35	60 g	22	8
Peanuts, roasted, salted	14	50 g	6	1
Pear, fresh	38	120 g	11	4
Pear halves, canned, in natural juice	44	120 g	13	5
Pear halves, canned, in reduced-sugar syrup	25	120 g	14	4
Pears, dried, ready to eat	43	60 g	27	12
Peas, green, frozen, boiled	48	80 g	7	3
Peas, yellow, split, dried, soaked overnight, boiled	25	150 g	85	21
Pecan nuts, raw	10	50 g	3	0
Pecans, raw	10	50 g	3	0
Pineapple, fresh	59	120 g	10	6
Pineapple juice, unsweetened	46	250 ml	34	16
Pitta bread, white, mini	68	30 g	15	10
Pitta bread, wholemeal	56	60 g	28	16
PIZZA				
Pizza Hut, Super Supreme, pan	36■	100 g	24	9
Pizza Hut, Super Supreme, thin and crispy	30■	100 g	22	7

FOOD	GI	NOMINAL SERVE SIZE	AVAILABLE CARB PER SERVE	GL PER SERVE
Pizza, Super Supreme, pan, Pizza Hut	36■	100 g	24	9
Pizza, Super Supreme, thin and crispy, Pizza Hut	30■	100 g	22	7
Plum, raw	39	120 g	12	5
Polenta, boiled	68	150 g	13	9
Polos®	70	30 g	30	21
Pop-Tarts™, chocotastic	70	50 g	36	25
Popcorn, plain, cooked in microwave	72	20 g	11	8
Pork	★■	120 g	0	0
Porridge oats, organic	63	50 g	29	18
Porridge oats, Scottish	63	50 g	31	20
Potato crisps, plain, salted	54■	50 g	18	10
POTATOES				
Desiree, peeled, boiled 35 mins	101	150 g	17	17
French fries, frozen, reheated in microwave	75■	150 g	29	22
Instant mashed potato	85	150 g	20	17
New, canned, microwaved 3 mins	65	150 g	18	12
New, unpeeled, boiled 20 mins	78	150 g	21	13
Sweet potato, baked	46	150 g	25	11
Pound cake, plain	54■	50 g	23	12
PRE-PACKED MEALS				
Beef and ale casserole, Tesco Finest	53	300 g	15	8

Pre-packed meals—Chicken korma and rice, Tesco Healthy Living

FOOD	GI	NOMINAL SERVE SIZE	AVAILABLE CARB PER SERVE	GL PER SERVE
Chicken korma and rice, Tesco Healthy Living	45	450 g	72	32
Chicken korma and peshwari rice, Tesco Finest	44	550 g	88	39
Chicken tikka masala and rice, Tesco Healthy Living	34	550 g	111	38
Cottage pie	65	500 g	56	36
Cumberland fish pie	40	250 g	26	10
Cumberland pie	29	500 g	62	18
Lamb moussaka, Tesco Finest	35	330 g	30	11
Lasagne, beef (frozen)	47	400 g	47	22
Lasagne, meat, chilled, Tesco Healthy Living	28	340 g	43	12
Lasagne, Tesco Finest	34	300 g	31	10
Mushroom stroganoff with rice	26	400 g	58	15
Sausage and mash	61	500 g	67	41
Shepherds pie	66	500 g	74	49
Steak and ale with cheddar mash, Tesco Finest	48	550 g	47	23
Tandoori chicken masala and rice, Tesco Finest	45	550 g	112	50
Pretzels, oven-baked, traditional wheat flavour	83	30 g	20	16
Probiotic drink, cranberry	56	100 ml	12	7
Probiotic drink, orange	30	100 ml	13	4
Probiotic drink, original	34	100 ml	12	4

★ little or no carbs ■ high in saturated fat

FOOD	GI	NOMINAL SERVE SIZE	AVAILABLE CARB PER SERVE	GL PER SERVE
Probiotic drink, pink grapefruit	60	100 ml	13	8
Probiotic yoghurt, prune	44	170 ml	24	11
Probiotic yoghurt, raspberry	45	170 ml	24	11
Probiotic yoghurt, strawberry	52	170 ml	24	13
Prunes, pitted	29	60 g	33	10
Puffed rice cakes, white	82	25 g	21	17
Puffed Wheat, breakfast cereal	80	30 g	21	17
PULSES				
Black beans, boiled	30	150 g	25	5
Black-eyed beans, soaked, boiled	42	150 g	29	12
Borlotti beans, canned, drained	41	75 g	12	5
Butter beans, canned, drained	36	75 g	12	4
Butter beans, dried, soaked overnight, boiled	26	150 g	75	19
Cannellini beans	31	85 g	12	4
Chickpeas, canned in brine	40	150 g	22	9
Chickpeas, dried, boiled	28	150 g	24	7
Four bean mix, canned, drained	37	75 g	12	5
Haricot beans, cooked, canned	38	150 g	31	12
Haricot beans, dried, boiled	33	150 g	31	10
Heinz® Baked Beans in tomato sauce, canned	49	150 g	17	8
Kidney beans, dark red, canned, drained	43	150 g	25	7

Pulses—Kidney beans, red

FOOD	GI	NOMINAL SERVE SIZE	AVAILABLE CARB PER SERVE	GL PER SERVE
Kidney beans, red, canned, drained	36	150 g	17	9
Kidney beans, red, dried, soaked overnight, boiled	51	150 g	60	31
Lentils, green, dried, boiled	30	150 g	17	5
Lentils, red, split, boiled	21	150 g	77	16
Lima beans, baby, frozen, reheated	32	150 g	30	10
Pearl barley, boiled	35	150 g	123	43
Peas, yellow, split, dried, soaked overnight, boiled	25	150 g	85	21
Soyabeans, canned	14	150 g	6	1
Soyabeans, dried, boiled	18	150 g	6	1
Pumpernickel bread	50	30 g	10	5
Pumpkin	75	80 g	4	3
Quinoa, organic, boiled	53	100 g	17	9
Radishes	★	15 g	0	0
Raisins	64	60 g	44	28
Raspberries	★	65 g	0	0
Ravioli, meat-filled, durum wheat flour, boiled	39■	180 g	38	15
Red kidney beans, dried, soaked overnight, boiled	51	150 g	60	31
Rhubarb	★	125 g	0	0
RICE				
Basmati rice, boiled, Tesco Value	52	75 g	40	21

FOOD	GI	NOMINAL SERVE SIZE	AVAILABLE CARB PER SERVE	GL PER SERVE
Basmati rice, Indian, boiled	69	75 g	57	39
Basmati rice, Indian, easy cook, boiled	67	75 g	60	40
Basmati rice, organic, boiled	57	75 g	57	33
Basmati rice, white, boiled	58	150 g	38	22
Glutinous rice, white, cooked in rice cooker	98	150 g	32	31
Instant rice, white, cooked 6 mins	87	150 g	42	36
Jasmine rice, white, long-grain, cooked in rice cooker	109	150 g	42	46
Risotto rice, Arborio, boiled	69	150 g	43	29
Wild rice, boiled	57	164 g	32	18
Rice cakes, puffed, white	82	25 g	21	17
Rice noodles, dried, boiled	61	176 g	39	24
Rice noodles, fresh, boiled	40	180 g	39	15
Rice pasta, brown, gluten-free, boiled	92	180 g	38	35
Rice vermicelli, dried, boiled	58	180 g	39	22
Risotto rice, Arborio, boiled	69	150 g	43	29
Roll (bread), white	73	30 g	16	12
Rye bread, wholemeal	51	40 g	13	7
Rye, grain	34	50 g	38	13
Salami	★■	120 g	0	0
Salmon, fresh or canned in water or brine	★	150 g	0	0

★ little or no carbs ■ high in saturated fat

FOOD	GI	NOMINAL SERVE SIZE	AVAILABLE CARB PER SERVE	GL PER SERVE
Sardines	★	60 g	0	0
Sausage and mash, pre-packed	61	500 g	67	41
Sausages, fried	28■	100 g	3	1
Scallops, natural, plain	★	160 g	0	0
Scones, plain, made from packet mix	92	25 g	9	8
SEAFOOD				
Calamari rings, squid, not battered or crumbed	★	70 g	0	0
Fish	★	120 g	0	0
Oysters, natural, plain	★	85 g	0	0
Salmon, fresh or canned in water or brine	★	150 g	0	0
Sardines	★	60 g	0	0
Scallops, natural, plain	★	160 g	0	0
Squid or calamari, not battered or crumbed	★	70 g	0	0
Sushi, salmon	48	100 g	36	17
Trout, fresh or frozen	★	63 g	0	0
Tuna, fresh or canned in water or brine	★	120 g	0	0
Semolina, cooked	55	150 g	11	6
Shallots	★	10 g	0	0
Shepherds pie, pre-packed	66	500 g	74	49
Shredded Wheat breakfast cereal	75	30 g	20	15

FOOD	GI	NOMINAL SERVE SIZE	AVAILABLE CARB PER SERVE	GL PER SERVE
Skimmed milk (0.1% fat)	32	250 ml	12	4
Skittles®	70■	50 g	45	32
SNACK FOODS				
Chicken nuggets, frozen, reheated in microwave 5 mins	46■	100 g	16	7
Chilli beef noodles, Tesco Finest	42	450 g	68	29
Chow mein, chicken (Serves One)	47	475 g	60	28
Chow mein, chicken, Tesco Healthy Living	55	450 g	34	19
Fajitas, chicken	42	275 g	39	17
Fish fingers	38■	100 g	19	7
French fries, frozen, reheated in microwave	75■	150 g	29	22
Heinz® Baked Beans in tomato sauce, canned	49	150 g	17	8
Jelly beans	78	30 g	28	22
Jelly, diet, made from crystals with water	★	125 g	0	0
Licorice, soft	78	60 g	42	33
M&M's®, peanut	33■	30 g	17	6
Mars Bar®, regular	62■	60 g	40	25
Marshmallows, plain, pink and white	62	25 g	20	12
Milky Bar®, plain white chocolate, Nestlé®	44■	50 g	29	13

Snack foods—Muesli bar, chewy, with choc chips or fruit

FOOD	GI	NOMINAL SERVE SIZE	AVAILABLE CARB PER SERVE	GL PER SERVE
Muesli bar, chewy, with choc chips or fruit	54■	31 g	21	12
Muesli bar, crunchy, with dried fruit	61	30 g	21	13
Peanuts, roasted, salted	14	50 g	6	1
Pizza Hut, Super Supreme, pan	36■	100 g	24	9
Pizza Hut, Super Supreme, thin and crispy	30■	100 g	22	7
Polos®	70	30 g	30	21
Pop-Tarts™, chocotastic	70	50 g	36	25
Popcorn, plain, cooked in microwave	72	20 g	11	8
Potato crisps, plain, salted	54■	50 g	18	10
Pretzels, oven-baked, traditional wheat flavour	83	30 g	20	16
Skittles®	70■	50 g	45	32
Sweet and sour chicken with noodles (Serves One)	41	475 g	82	33
Taco shells, cornmeal-based, baked	68	20 g	12	8
Twix® bar	44■	60 g	39	17
SOFT DRINKS				
Coca-Cola®, soft drink	53	250 ml	26	14
Diet soft drinks	★	250 ml	0	0
Fanta®, orange soft drink	68	250 ml	34	23
SOUPS				
Black bean soup, canned	64	250 ml	27	17

★ little or no carbs ■ high in saturated fat

Soups—Consommé, clear, chicken or vegetable

FOOD	GI	NOMINAL SERVE SIZE	AVAILABLE CARB PER SERVE	GL PER SERVE
Consommé, clear, chicken or vegetable	★	205 ml	2	0
Green pea soup, canned	66	250 ml	41	27
Lentil soup, canned	44	250 ml	21	9
Minestrone soup, traditional, canned	39	250 ml	18	7
Split pea soup, canned	60	250 ml	27	16
Tomato soup, canned	45	250 ml	17	6
Sourdough bread, organic, stoneground, wholemeal	59	32 g	12	7
Sourdough rye bread	48	30 g	12	6
Sourdough wheat bread	54	30 g	14	8
Soy and Linseed bread, Bürgen®	55	70 g	24	13
Soyabeans, canned	14	150 g	6	1
Soyabeans, dried, boiled	18	150 g	6	1
Soya milk, calcium-enriched	36	250 ml	18	6
Soya milk, low fat, calcium-fortified	44	250 ml	17	8
SOYA MILK				
Soya milk, calcium-enriched	36	250 ml	18	6
Soya milk, low fat, calcium-fortified	44	250 ml	17	8
SOYA PRODUCTS				
Soyabeans, canned	14	150 g	6	1
Soyabeans, dried, boiled	18	150 g	6	1
Soya yoghurt, peach and mango, 2% fat	50	200 g	26	13

★ little or no carbs ■ high in saturated fat

Soya products—Tofu (bean curd), plain, unsweetened

FOOD	GI	NOMINAL SERVE SIZE	AVAILABLE CARB PER SERVE	GL PER SERVE
Tofu (bean curd), plain, unsweetened	★	100 g	0	0
Spaghetti, gluten-free, rice and split pea, canned in tomato sauce	68	220 g	27	19
Spaghetti, white, durum wheat, boiled 10–15 mins	44	180 g	48	21
Spaghetti, wholemeal, boiled	42	180 g	42	16
Special K®, regular, breakfast cereal, Kellogg's®	56	30 g	21	11
Spinach	★	75 g	0	0
Spirali pasta, white, durum wheat, boiled	43	180 g	44	19
Split pea soup, canned	60	250 ml	27	16
Sponge cake, plain, unfilled	46■	63 g	36	17
SPORTS DRINKS				
Isostar® sports drink	70	250 ml	18	13
Lucozade®, original, sparkling glucose drink	95	250 ml	42	40
SPREADS				
Golden syrup	63	20 g	17	11
Hommous, regular	6	30 g	5	1
Maple syrup, pure, Canadian	54	24 g	18	10
Nutella®, hazelnut spread	33	20 g	12	4
Strawberry jam, regular	51	30 g	20	10
Spring onions	★	15 g	0	0

FOOD	GI	NOMINAL SERVE SIZE	AVAILABLE CARB PER SERVE	GL PER SERVE
Squash, yellow	★	70 g	0	0
Squid or calamari, not battered or crumbed	★	70 g	0	0
Steak and ale with cheddar mash, pre-packed, Tesco Finest	48	550 g	47	23
Steak, any cut	★■	120 g	0	0
Strawberries, fresh	40	120 g	3	1
Strawberry jam, regular	51	30 g	20	10
Sugar	68	10 g	10	7
Sultana Bran™, breakfast cereal, Kellogg's®	73	30 g	19	14
Sultanas	58	60 g	42	24
Sultanas, Tesco Value	56	60 g	42	24
Sushi, salmon	48	100 g	36	17
Swede, cooked	72	150 g	10	7
Sweetcorn, on the cob, boiled	48	80 g	16	8
Sweetcorn, whole kernel, canned, drained	46	80 g	14	7
Sweetened condensed full fat milk	61■	50 g	28	17
Sweetened dried cranberries	64	40 g	29	19
Taco shells, cornmeal-based, baked	68	20 g	12	8
Tagliatelle, egg, dry pasta, boiled	46	50 g	33	15
TESCO BREADS				
Crusty malted wheat bread, Tesco Finest	52	30 g	13	7

★ little or no carbs ■ high in saturated fat

FOOD	GI	NOMINAL SERVE SIZE	AVAILABLE CARB PER SERVE	GL PER SERVE
Fruit and cinnamon bread, Tesco Finest	71	37 g	20	14
Fruit loaf, Tesco Value	90	30 g	18	16
Pitta bread, white, Tesco Value	69	60 g	31	21
TESCO BREAKFAST CEREALS				
Branflakes, Tesco Healthy Living	50	30 g	20	10
Fruit and fibre cereal, Tesco Value	68	40 g	26	18
Muesli, Tesco Healthy Eating	86	50 g	36	31
Muesli, Tesco Value	64	50 g	31	20
Porridge oats, Tesco Value	63	50 g	30	19
Sultana bran, Tesco Healthy Living	90	30 g	17	16
Tofu (bean curd), plain, unsweetened	★	100 g	0	0
Tomato	★	150 g	0	0
Tomato juice, no added sugar	38	250 ml	9	4
Tomato soup, canned	45	250 ml	17	6
Tortellini, cheese, boiled	50■	180 g	21	10
Trout, fresh or frozen	★	63 g	0	0
Tuna, fresh or canned in water or brine	★	120 g	0	0
Turkey	★■	140 g	0	0
Twix® bar	44■	60 g	39	17
2 minute noodles, 99% fat free, Maggi	71	75	51	34
2 minute noodles, regular, Maggi	54	75	51	34

Vanilla cake made from packet mix with vanilla frosting

FOOD	GI	NOMINAL SERVE SIZE	AVAILABLE CARB PER SERVE	GL PER SERVE
Vanilla cake made from packet mix with vanilla frosting,	42■	111 g	58	24
Vanilla custard, reduced fat	37	100 ml	15	6
Vanilla ice-cream, full fat	38■	50 g	9	3
Veal	★	120 g	0	0
VEGETABLES				
Artichokes, globe, fresh or canned in brine	★	80 g	0	0
Arugula	★	30 g	0	0
Asparagus	★	100 g	0	0
Aubergine	★	100 g	0	0
Bean sprouts, raw	★	14 g	0	0
Beetroot, canned	64	80 g	7	5
Bok choy	★	100 g	0	0
Broad beans	79	80 g	11	9
Broccoli	★	60 g	0	0
Brussels sprouts	★	100 g	0	0
Cabbage	★	70 g	0	0
Carrots, peeled, boiled	41	80 g	5	2
Cauliflower	★	60 g	0	0
Celery	★	40 g	0	0
Chillies, fresh or dried	★	20 g	0	0
Chives, fresh	★	4 g	0	0
Courgette	★	100 g	0	0

FOOD	GI	NOMINAL SERVE SIZE	AVAILABLE CARB PER SERVE	GL PER SERVE
Cucumber	★	45 g	0	0
Desiree potato, peeled, boiled 35 mins	101	150 g	17	17
Endive	★	30 g	0	0
Fennel	★	90 g	0	0
Garlic	★	5 g	0	0
Ginger	★	10 g	0	0
Green beans	★	70 g	0	0
Herbs, fresh or dried	★	2 g	0	0
Leeks	★	80 g	0	0
Lettuce	★	50 g	0	0
Mung beans	39	150 g	17	5
Mushrooms	★	35 g	0	0
New potato, canned, microwaved 3 mins	65	150 g	18	12
New potato, unpeeled and boiled 20 mins	78	150 g	21	13
Okra	★	80 g	0	0
Onions, raw, peeled	★	30 g	0	0
Parsnips	97	80 g	12	12
Peas, dried, boiled	22	150 g	9	2
Peas, green, frozen, boiled	48	80 g	7	3
Pumpkin	75	80 g	4	3
Radishes	★	15 g	0	0

★ little or no carbs ■ high in saturated fat

FOOD	GI	NOMINAL SERVE SIZE	AVAILABLE CARB PER SERVE	GL PER SERVE
Shallots	★	10 g	0	0
Spinach	★	75 g	0	0
Spring onions	★	15 g	0	0
Squash, yellow	★	70 g	0	0
Swede, cooked	72	150 g	10	7
Sweetcorn, on the cob, boiled	48	80 g	16	8
Sweetcorn, whole kernel, canned, drained	46	80 g	14	7
Tomato	★	150 g	0	0
Watercress	★	8 g	0	0
Yam, peeled, boiled	37	150 g	36	13
Vermicelli, white, durum wheat, boiled	35	180 g	44	16
Vinegar	★	5 ml	0	0
Vogel's Honey and Oat Bran bread	49	40g	13	7
Wafer biscuits, vanilla, plain	77■	25 g	18	14
Water crackers, plain	78	25 g	18	14
Watercress	★	8 g	0	0
Watermelon, raw	76	120 g	6	4
Wheat, cracked, bulgur, ready to eat	48	150 g	26	12
WHITE BREAD				
Pitta bread, white, mini	57	30 g	17	10
Pitta bread, white, Tesco Value	69	60 g	31	21

★ little or no carbs ■ high in saturated fat

W

Y

FOOD	GI	NOMINAL SERVE SIZE	AVAILABLE CARB PER SERVE	GL PER SERVE
Roll (bread), white	73	30 g	16	12
White bread, regular, sliced	71	30 g	14	10
White bread, regular, sliced	71	30 g	14	10
WHOLEMEAL BREAD				
Pitta bread, wholemeal	56	60 g	28	16
Rye bread, wholemeal	51	40 g	13	7
Sourdough bread, organic, stoneground, wholemeal	59	32 g	12	7
Wild rice, boiled	57	164 g	32	18
Yam, peeled, boiled	37	150 g	36	13
YOGHURT				
Fat-free yoghurts, various flavours	40	200 g	31	12
Greek style, honey topped	36	140 g	19	7
Low fat, apricot	42	150 g	21	9
Low fat, black cherry	41	150 g	22	9
Low fat, hazelnut	53	150 g	21	11
Low fat, natural	35	200 g	12	4
Low fat, raspberry	34	150 g	22	8
Low fat, strawberry	62	150 g	22	13
Low fat, toffee	51	150 g	26	13
Tesco Finest, black cherry	17	150 g	24	4
Tesco Finest, bourbon vanilla	64	150 g	29	18
Tesco Finest, champagne rhubarb	49	150 g	25	12

FOOD	GI	NOMINAL SERVE SIZE	AVAILABLE CARB PER SERVE	GL PER SERVE
Tesco Finest, creme fraiche dessert, peach	28	150 g	23	7
Tesco Finest, creme fraiche dessert, raspberry	30	150 g	17	5
Tesco Finest, Devonshire fudge	37	150 g	34	12
Tesco Finest, lemon curd	67	150 g	30	20
Tesco Finest, orange blossom	42	150 g	30	13
Tesco Finest, Scottish raspberry	32	150 g	28	9
Tesco Finest, strawberry and cream	41	150 g	23	8
Tesco Finest, Valencia orange	34	150 g	25	13
Tesco Finest, white peach	54	150 g	24	13
Tesco Healthy Living, fromage frais, blackcurrant	22	100 g	7	2
Tesco Healthy Living, fromage frais, mango and papaya	25	100 g	7	2
Tesco Healthy Living, fromage frais, passionfruit and pineapple	18	100 g	7	1
Tesco Healthy Living, fromage frais, peach and apricot	22	100 g	7	1
Tesco Healthy Living, fromage frais, raspberry	31	100 g	7	2
Tesco Healthy Living, fromage frais, red cherry	25	100 g	7	2
Tesco Healthy Living, fromage frais, strawberry	29	100 g	7	2
Tesco Healthy Living, fromage frais, mandarin and orange	19	100 g	7	1

★ little or no carbs ■ high in saturated fat

FOOD	GI	NOMINAL SERVE SIZE	AVAILABLE CARB PER SERVE	GL PER SERVE
Tesco Healthy Living Light, apricot	11	125 g	8	1
Tesco Healthy Living Light, black cherry	67	200 g	17	12
Tesco Healthy Living Light, guava and passionfruit	24	125 g	8	2
Tesco Healthy Living Light, mango	32	125 g	8	3
Tesco Healthy Living Light, morello cherry	35	125 g	8	3
Tesco Healthy Living Light, peach and apricot	28	200 g	16	5
Tesco Healthy Living Light, peach and vanilla	26	125 g	8	2
Tesco Healthy Living Light, pineapple	38	125 g	8	3
Tesco Healthy Living Light, raspberry	43	200 g	16	7
Tesco Healthy Living Light, raspberry	28	125 g	8	2
Tesco Healthy Living Light, raspberry and cranberry	42	125 g	8	3
Tesco Healthy Living Light, raspberry and black cherry	37	125 g	8	3
Tesco Healthy Living Light, strawberry	30	200 g	16	5
Tesco Healthy Living Light, toffee	41	200 g	15	6
Tesco Healthy Living Light, vanilla	47	200 g	14	7
Tesco Value, low fat, peach melba	56	125 g	18	10
Tesco Value, low fat, strawberry	85	125 g	18	15

FOOD	GI	NOMINAL SERVE SIZE	AVAILABLE CARB PER SERVE	GL PER SERVE
Tesco Value, peach melba	57	125 g	20	11
Yoghurt, diet, low fat, no added sugar, vanilla or fruit (averaged)	20	200 g	13	3

Low to High
GI Values

These tables are designed to enable you to make easy and effective substitutions to what you currently eat, to help you lower the GI of your diet as a whole.

Low GI: 55 or under
Medium GI: 56-69
High GI: 70 or over

With this quick reference guide you can select the lower GI varieties in each food category. The foods are listed in three columns: low, medium and high.

The food categories include:

Bakery products	85
Beverages	86
Biscuits	87
Bread	88
Breakfast cereal bars	89
Breakfast cereals	90

Cakes	92
Cereal grains	93
Chocolate	94
Crackers and crispbreads	95
Dairy products	96
Fruit and vegetable juice	97
Fruit – canned	98
– dried	99
– fresh	100
Meat	101
Milk	102
Muffins	103
Noodles	104
Nuts	105
Pasta	106
Pizza	109
Potatoes	110
Pre-packed meals	111
Pulses	113
Rice	116
Seafood	117
Snack foods	118
Soft drinks	120
Soups	121
Soya milk	122
Soya products	123
Sports drinks	124
Spreads	125
Vegetables	126

White bread   129

Wholemeal bread   130

Yoghurt   131

Key

■ Means that a food may be high in saturated fat.
   As we have mentioned previously, the GI should
   not be used in isolation, but the overall nutritional
   value of the food needs to be considered.

BAKERY PRODUCTS

LOW	MEDIUM	HIGH
	Croissant, plain ■	Bagel, white
	Crumpet, white	Scones, plain, made from packet mix

BEVERAGES

LOW	MEDIUM	HIGH
Probiotic drink, orange	Probiotic drink, cranberry	
Probiotic drink, original	Probiotic drink, pink grapefruit	
Probiotic yoghurt, prune		
Probiotic yoghurt, raspberry		
Probiotic yoghurt, strawberry		

BISCUITS

LOW	MEDIUM	HIGH
Rich Tea® biscuits ■	Digestive biscuits, plain ■ Oatcakes ■ Shortbread, plain ■	Wafer biscuits, vanilla, plain ■

BREAD

LOW	MEDIUM	HIGH
Crusty malted wheat bread, Tesco Finest	Fruit loaf, sliced	Black rye bread
Fruit & Muesli loaf, Bürgen®	Hamburger bun, white	Dark rye bread
Fruit loaf, thick sliced	Light rye bread	Fruit and cinnamon bread, Tesco Finest
Pumpernickel bread	Malt loaf, organic	Fruit loaf, Tesco Value
Rye bread, wholemeal	Multi-grain batch bread	Melba toast, plain
Sourdough rye bread	Multigrain sandwich bread	Roll (bread), white
Sourdough wheat bread	Oatmeal batch bread	White bread, regular, sliced
Soya and Linseed, Bürgen®	Pitta bread, white	
Vogel's Honey and Oat Bran bread	Pitta bread, white, mini	
	Pitta bread, white, Tesco Value	
	Pitta bread, wholemeal	
	Sourdough bread, organic, stoneground, wholemeal	

BREAKFAST CEREAL BARS

LOW	MEDIUM	HIGH
		Crunchy Nut Corn Flakes Bar, Kellogg's®

BREAKFAST CEREALS

LOW	MEDIUM	HIGH
All-Bran®, Kellogg's®	Fruit and fibre breakfast cereal	Bran Flakes, Kellogg's®
Branflakes, Tesco Healthy Living	Fruit and fibre cereal, Tesco Value	Coco Pops®, Kellogg's®
Frosties®, Kellogg's®	Muesli, fruit	Corn Flakes®, Kellogg's®
Hi fibre bran cereal	Muesli, fruit and nut	Crunchy Nut Corn Flakes, Kellogg's®
Oat bran, raw, unprocessed	Muesli, Tesco Value	Muesli, Tesco Healthy Eating
Semolina, cooked	Muesli, wholewheat	Porridge, instant, made with water
	Oats, rolled, raw	Puffed Wheat
	Porridge oats, organic	Rice Krispies®, Kellogg's®
	Porridge oats, Scottish	Shredded Wheat
	Porridge oats, Tesco Value	
	Special K®, regular, Kellogg's®	

BREAKFAST CEREALS (cont.)

LOW	MEDIUM	HIGH
		Sultana bran, Tesco Healthy Living
		Sultana Bran™, Kellogg's®

CAKES

LOW	MEDIUM	HIGH
Banana cake, home-made ■	Angel food cake, plain ■	Cupcake, strawberry-iced ■
Chocolate cake, made from packet mix with icing ■		
Pound cake, plain ■		
Sponge cake, plain, unfilled ■		
Vanilla cake made from packet mix with vanilla frosting ■		

CEREAL GRAINS

LOW	MEDIUM	HIGH
Barley, pearled, boiled	Buckwheat, puffed	
Buckwheat, boiled	Cornmeal (polenta), boiled	
Bulgur, cracked wheat, ready to eat	Couscous, boiled 5 mins	
Quinoa, organic, boiled	Polenta, boiled	
Rye, grain		
Semolina, cooked		

CHOCOLATE

LOW	MEDIUM	HIGH
Chocolate cake, made from packet mix with icing ■	Mars Bar®, regular ■	
Chocolate, dark, plain ■		
Chocolate, milk, plain, Cadbury's® ■		
Chocolate, white, plain, Nestlé® ■		
M&M's®, peanut ■		
Milky Bar®, plain white chocolate, Nestlé® ■		
Twix® bar ■		

CRACKERS AND CRISPBREADS

LOW	MEDIUM	HIGH
		Melba toast, plain
		Rice cakes, puffed, white
		Water crackers, plain

DAIRY PRODUCTS

LOW	MEDIUM	HIGH
Cheese ■		
Custard, home-made from milk, wheat starch and sugar ■		
Vanilla custard, reduced fat		

FRUIT AND VEGETABLE JUICE

LOW	MEDIUM	HIGH
Apple juice, no added sugar		
Carrot juice, freshly made		
Cranberry Juice Cocktail, Ocean Spray		
Granny Smith apple juice, unsweetened		
Grapefruit juice, unsweetened		
Orange juice, unsweetened		
Pineapple juice, unsweetened		
Tomato juice, no added sugar		

FRUIT, CANNED

LOW	MEDIUM	HIGH
Peaches in natural juice	Apricots in light syrup	Lychees in syrup, drained
Pear halves in natural juice	Peaches in heavy syrup	
Pear halves in reduced-sugar syrup	Peaches in light syrup	

FRUIT, DRIED

LOW	MEDIUM	HIGH
Apple	Cranberries, sweetened	Dates
Apricots, ready to eat	Figs, tenderised	
Apricots, ready to eat, bite size	Mixed fruit, Tesco Value	
Dates, Arabic, vacuum-packed	Raisins	
Peaches, ready to eat	Sultanas	
Pears, ready to eat	Sultanas, Tesco Value	
Prunes, pitted		

FRUIT, FRESH

LOW	MEDIUM	HIGH
Apple	Apricots	Watermelon
Avocado	Cantaloupe	
Banana	Cherries, dark	
Custard apple, flesh only	Paw paw	
Grapefruit	Pineapple	
Grapes		
Kiwi fruit		
Lemon		
Lime		
Mango		
Orange		
Peach		
Pear		
Plum		
Raspberries		
Rhubarb		
Strawberries		

MEAT

LOW	MEDIUM	HIGH
Bacon		
Beef ■		
Brawn ■		
Chicken		
Duck ■		
Ham, leg or shoulder ■		
Lamb		
Liver sausage ■		
Pork ■		
Salami ■		
Sausages, fried ■		
Steak, any cut ■		
Turkey ■		
Veal		

MILK

LOW	MEDIUM	HIGH
Semi-skimmed (1.4% fat)	Condensed, sweetened, full fat ■	
Skimmed (0.1% fat)		
Semi-skimmed, pasteurised, British, Dairycrest		
Semi-skimmed, pasteurised, organic, Arla		
Skimmed, pasteurised, British, Dairycrest		
Standardised homogenised, pasteurised, British, Dairycrest		
Whole, pasteurised, fresh, organic, Arla		

MUFFINS

LOW	MEDIUM	HIGH
Apple muffin, home-made ■	Blueberry muffin, commercially made ■	
	Bran muffin, commercially made ■	

NOODLES

LOW	MEDIUM	HIGH
Bean thread noodles, dried, boiled	Instant noodles, 99% fat free	2 minute noodles, 99% fat free, Maggi
Instant noodles, regular ■	Rice noodles, dried, boiled	
Mung bean noodles (bean thread), dried, boiled	Rice vermicelli, dried, boiled	
Rice noodles, fresh, boiled		
2 minute noodles, regular, Maggi		

NUTS

LOW	MEDIUM	HIGH
Cashew nut halves		
Cashew nuts		
Cashew nuts, organic, roasted and salted		
Cashew nuts, roasted and salted		
Fruit and nut mix, Tesco Finest		
Mixed nuts and raisins		
Mixed nuts, roasted and salted		
Peanuts, roasted, salted		
Pecan nuts, raw		
Tropical fruit and nut mix, Tesco Finest		

PASTA

LOW	MEDIUM	HIGH
Cannelloni, spinach and ricotta	Gnocchi, cooked	Rice pasta, brown, boiled
Fettuccine, egg, cooked	Spaghetti, gluten-free, rice and split pea, canned in tomato sauce	Rice pasta, brown, gluten-free, boiled
Fusilli pasta twists, dry pasta, boiled		
Fusilli pasta twists, tricolour, dry pasta, boiled		
Fusilli pasta twists, wholewheat, dry pasta, boiled		
Lasagne		
Lasagne sheets, dry pasta, boiled, Tesco Value		
Lasagne, egg, dry pasta, boiled		
Lasagne, egg, verdi, dry pasta, boiled		

LOW	MEDIUM	HIGH
Lasagne, vegetarian		
Linguine, thick, durum wheat, boiled		
Linguine, thin, durum wheat, boiled		
Macaroni, white, plain, boiled		
Pasta bake, tomato and mozzarella		
Ravioli, meat-filled, durum wheat flour, boiled ∎		
Spaghetti, white, durum wheat, boiled 10–15 mins		
Spaghetti, wholemeal, boiled		

PASTA (cont)

LOW	MEDIUM	HIGH
Spirali, white, durum wheat, boiled		
Tagliatelle, egg, dry pasta, boiled		
Tortellini, cheese, boiled ■		
Vermicelli, white, durum wheat, boiled		

PIZZA

LOW	MEDIUM\	HIGH
Pizza Hut, Super Supreme, pan ■		
Pizza Hut, Super Supreme, thin and crispy ■		

POTATOES

LOW	MEDIUM	HIGH
Sweet potato, baked	New, canned, microwaved 3 mins	Desiree, peeled, boiled 35 mins
		French fries, frozen, reheated in microwave ■
		Instant mashed potato
		New, unpeeled, boiled 20 mins

PRE-PACKED MEALS

LOW	MEDIUM	HIGH
Beef and ale casserole, Tesco Finest	Cottage pie	
Chicken korma and peshwari rice, Tesco Finest	Sausage and mash	
Chicken korma and rice, Tesco Healthy Living	Shepherds pie	
Chicken tikka masala and rice, Tesco Healthy Living		
Cumberland fish pie		
Cumberland pie		
Lamb moussaka, Tesco Finest		
Lasagne, beef (frozen)		
Lasagne, meat, chilled, Tesco Healthy Living		

LOW	MEDIUM	HIGH
Lasagne, Tesco Finest		
Mushroom stroganoff with rice		
Steak and ale with cheddar mash, Tesco Finest		
Tandoori chicken masala and rice, Tesco Finest		

PULSES

LOW	MEDIUM	HIGH
Black beans, boiled		
Black-eyed beans, soaked, boiled		
Borlotti beans, canned, drained		
Butter beans, canned, drained		
Butter beans, dried, soaked overnight, boiled		
Cannellini beans		
Chickpeas, canned in brine		
Chickpeas, dried, boiled		
Four bean mix, canned, drained		
Haricot beans, cooked, canned		
Haricot beans, dried, boiled		

PULSES (cont)

LOW	MEDIUM	HIGH
Heinz® Baked Beans in tomato sauce, canned		
Kidney beans, dark red, canned, drained		
Kidney beans, red, canned, drained		
Kidney beans, red, dried, soaked overnight, boiled		
Lentils, green, dried, boiled		
Lentils, red, split, boiled		
Lima beans, baby, frozen, reheated		
Pearl barley, boiled		
Peas, yellow, split, dried, soaked overnight, boiled		

PULSES (cont)

LOW	MEDIUM	HIGH
Soyabeans, canned		
Soyabeans, dried, boiled		

RICE

LOW	MEDIUM	HIGH
Basmati, boiled, Tesco Value	Basmati, Indian, boiled	Glutinous, white, cooked in rice cooker
	Basmati, Indian, easy cook, boiled	Instant, white, cooked 6 mins
	Basmati, organic, boiled	Jasmine, white, long-grain, cooked in rice cooker
	Basmati, white, boiled	
	Risotto, Arborio, boiled	
	Wild, boiled	

SEAFOOD

LOW	MEDIUM	HIGH
Calamari rings, squid, not battered or crumbed		
Fish		
Oysters, natural, plain		
Salmon, fresh or canned in water or brine		
Sardines		
Scallops, natural, plain		
Squid or calamari, not battered or crumbed		
Sushi, salmon		
Trout, fresh or frozen		
Tuna, fresh or canned in water or brine		

SNACK FOODS

LOW	MEDIUM	HIGH
Chicken nuggets, frozen, reheated in microwave 5 mins ■	Mars Bar®, regular ■	French fries, frozen, reheated in microwave ■
Chilli beef noodles, Tesco Finest	Marshmallows, plain, pink and white	Jelly beans
Chow mein, chicken (Serves One)	Muesli bar, crunchy, with dried fruit	Licorice, soft
		Polos®
Chow mein, chicken, Tesco Healthy Living	Taco shells, cornmeal-based, baked	Pop-Tarts™, chocotastic
Fajitas, chicken		Popcorn, plain, cooked in microwave
Fish fingers ■		Pretzels, oven-baked, traditional wheat flavour
Heinz® Baked Beans in tomato sauce, canned		Skittles® ■
Jelly, diet, made from crystals with water		
M&M's®, peanut ■		

LOW	MEDIUM	HIGH
Milky Bar®, plain white chocolate, Nestlé® ■		
Muesli bar, chewy, with choc chips or fruit ■		
Peanuts, roasted, salted		
Pizza Hut, Super Supreme, pan ■		
Pizza Hut, Super Supreme, thin and crispy ■		
Potato crisps, plain, salted ■		
Sweet and sour chicken with noodles (Serves One)		
Twix® bar ■		

SOFT DRINKS

LOW	MEDIUM	HIGH
Coca-Cola®, soft drink	Fanta®, orange soft drink	
Diet soft drinks		

SOUPS

LOW	MEDIUM	HIGH
Consommé, clear, chicken or vegetable ★	Black bean, canned	
Lentil, canned	Green pea, canned	
Minestrone, traditional, canned	Split pea, canned	
Tomato, canned		

SOYA MILK

LOW	MEDIUM	HIGH
Calcium-enriched		
Low fat, calcium-fortified		

SOYA PRODUCTS

LOW	MEDIUM	HIGH
Soyabeans, canned		
Soyabeans, dried, boiled		
Soya yoghurt, Peach and Mango, 2% fat		
Tofu (bean curd), plain, unsweetened ★		

SPORTS DRINKS

LOW	MEDIUM	HIGH
		Isostar® sports drink
		Lucozade®, original, sparkling glucose drink

SPREADS

LOW	MEDIUM	HIGH
Hommous, regular	Golden syrup	
Maple syrup, pure, Canadian		
Nutella®, hazelnut spread		
Strawberry jam, regular		

VEGETABLES

LOW	MEDIUM	HIGH
Artichokes, globe, fresh or canned in brine	Beetroot, canned	Broad beans
Arugula	New potato, canned, microwaved 3 mins	Desiree potato, peeled, boiled 35 mins
Asparagus		New potato, unpeeled and boiled 20 mins
Aubergine		Parsnips
Bean sprouts, raw		Pumpkin
Bok choy		Swede, cooked
Broccoli		
Brussels sprouts		
Cabbage		
Carrots, peeled, boiled		
Cauliflower		
Celery		
Chillies, fresh or dried		
Chives, fresh		

VEGETABLES

LOW	MEDIUM	HIGH
Courgette		
Cucumber		
Endive		
Fennel		
Garlic		
Ginger		
Green beans		
Herbs, fresh or dried		
Leeks		
Lettuce		
Mung beans		
Mushrooms		
Okra		
Onions, raw, peeled		
Peas, dried, boiled		
Peas, green, frozen, boiled		

VEGETABLES

LOW	MEDIUM	HIGH
Radishes		
Shallots		
Spinach		
Spring onions		
Squash, yellow		
Sweetcorn, on the cob, boiled		
Sweetcorn, whole kernel, canned, drained		
Tomato		
Watercress		
Yam, peeled, boiled		

WHITE BREAD

LOW	MEDIUM	HIGH
	Pitta bread, white, mini	Roll (bread), white
	Pitta bread, white, Tesco Value	White bread, regular, sliced

WHOLEMEAL BREAD

LOW	MEDIUM	HIGH
Rye bread, wholemeal	Pitta bread, wholemeal	
	Sourdough bread, organic, stoneground, wholemeal	

YOGHURT

LOW	MEDIUM	HIGH
Fat-free yoghurts, various flavours	Low fat, strawberry	Tesco Value, low fat, strawberry
Greek style, honey topped	Tesco Finest, bourbon vanilla	
Low fat, apricot	Tesco Finest, lemon curd	
Low fat, black cherry	Tesco Healthy Living Light, black cherry	
Low fat, hazelnut	Tesco Value, low fat, peach melba	
Low fat, natural	Tesco Value, peach melba	
Low fat, raspberry		
Low fat, toffee		
Tesco Finest, black cherry		
Tesco Finest, champagne rhubarb		
Tesco Finest, creme fraiche dessert, peach		

YOGHURT (cont)

LOW	MEDIUM	HIGH
Tesco Finest, creme fraiche dessert, raspberry		
Tesco Finest, Devonshire fudge		
Tesco Finest, orange blossom		
Tesco Finest, Scottish raspberry		
Tesco Finest, strawberry and cream		
Tesco Finest, Valencia orange		
Tesco Finest, white peach		
Tesco Healthy Living Light, apricot		

YOGHURT (cont)

LOW	MEDIUM	HIGH
Tesco Healthy Living Light, guava and passionfruit		
Tesco Healthy Living Light, mango		
Tesco Healthy Living Light, morello cherry		
Tesco Healthy Living Light, peach and apricot		
Tesco Healthy Living Light, peach and vanilla		
Tesco Healthy Living Light, pineapple		
Tesco Healthy Living Light, raspberry		

LOW	MEDIUM	HIGH
Tesco Healthy Living Light, raspberry and black cherry		
Tesco Healthy Living Light, raspberry and cranberry		
Tesco Healthy Living Light, strawberry		
Tesco Healthy Living Light, toffee		
Tesco Healthy Living Light, vanilla		
Tesco Healthy Living, fromage frais, passionfruit and pineapple		
Tesco Healthy Living, fromage frais, mandarin and orange		

LOW	MEDIUM	HIGH
Tesco Healthy Living, fromage frais, mango and papaya		
Tesco Healthy Living, fromage frais, peach and apricot		
Tesco Healthy Living, fromage frais, raspberry		
Tesco Healthy Living, fromage frais, red cherry		
Tesco Healthy Living, fromage frais, blackcurrant		
Tesco Healthy Living, fromage frais, strawberry		

LOW	MEDIUM	HIGH
Yoghurt, diet, low fat, no added sugar, vanilla or fruit (averaged)		
Yoghurt, Ski™, low fat, with sugar, Strawberry